FITNESS BOXING

THE ULTIMATE WORKOUT

C1 844290 60

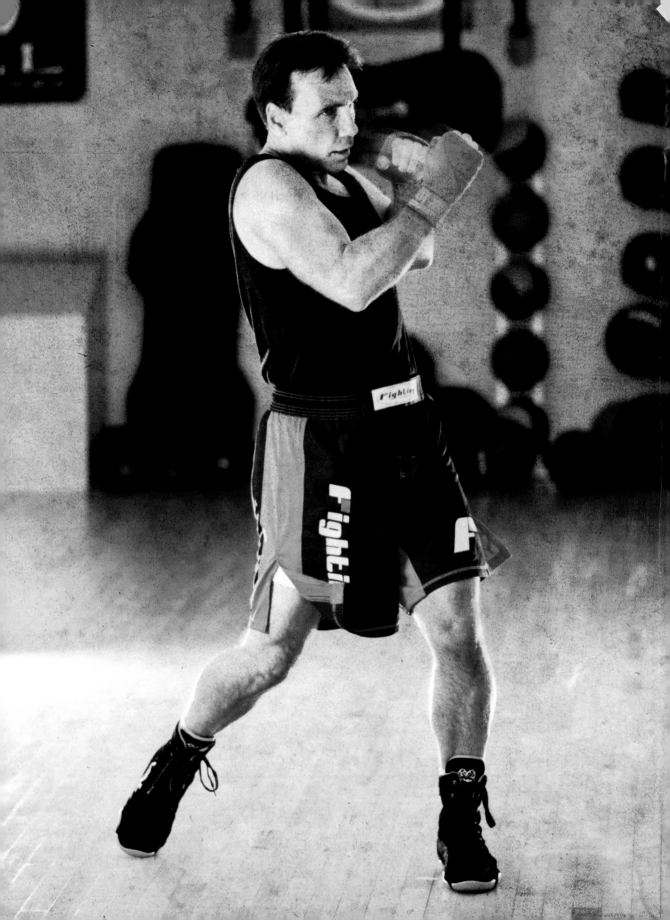

FITNESS BOXING

THE ULTIMATE WORKOUT

ANDY DUMAS & JAMIE DUMAS

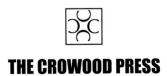

THE CROWOOD PRESS

First published in 2014 by
The Crowood Press Ltd
Ramsbury, Marlborough
Wiltshire SN8 2HR

www.crowood.com

© Andy Dumas and Jamie Du[...]

British Library Cataloguing-in-Publication Data
A catalogue record for this book is available from the British Library.

ISBN 978 1 84797 812 7

Dedication
Dedicated to our parents, Eve and Cliff Dumas Sr., and Joyce and Joseph Lipton

Acknowledgements
Our thanks go to Sergio Martinez, Floyd Mayweather Jr, Jose Sulaiman and Mauricio Sulaiman of the World Boxing Council; Jill Diamond, WBC female championship committee; Cecilia Brækhus and Greg Post; the team from Prime Time Personal Fitness & Boxing; Russ Anber, Julia Smith and everyone at Rival Boxing; Jeff McCarrol and Gabriella Ralph of the Ontario Racquet Club. We are also grateful to our photographers: Nikola Novak and Naoki Fakuda, Tanya Caruana, Leandro Almanzor Dumlao, David Hart, Andrew Finnigan, Donovan Irving, Angie LaFontaine, Kyla McCall and Ryan Moore.

Photo Credits
Cover photographs and instructional photographs by Nikola Novak (www.nikpix.ca).
Boxing champion photographs by Naoki Fakuda (www.naopix.com).
Additional photographs by Andy Dumas, Jamie Dumas (www.andydumas.ca) and Kyla McCall.

Disclaimer
Please note that the authors and the publisher of this book, and those others who have contributed to it, are not responsible in any manner whatsoever for any damage or injury of any kind that may result from practising, or applying, the principles, ideas, techniques and/or following the instructions/information described in this publication. Since the physical activities described in this book may be too strenuous in nature for some readers to engage in safely, it is essential that a doctor be consulted before participating.

Also by Andy Dumas and Jamie Dumas: *The One-Two Punch Boxing Workout, Knockout Fitness, Old School Boxing Fitness* and *Successful Boxing*.

Typeset by Andrew Finnigan, Waterdown, Ontario, Canada
Printed and bound in Singapore by Craft Print International

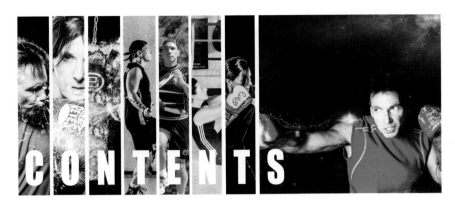

CONTENTS

FOREWORD

When I was growing up in Argentina, boxing was almost a religion in my home. Every time there was a fight, my family and friends would get together at my house and watch the match. My work ethic and determination served me well in sport: as a soccer player, as an award-winning cyclist, and as a tennis player who relished the one-on-one competition. In these sports I would out-think and out-work my competitors. Then when I was twenty years old I found boxing. There was something deep inside that told me I would be successful at it, and on my second day in the boxing gym I knew in my heart and soul that I would be a world champion one day.

Although much of a boxer's workout regimen is based on old-style training, boxers these days are better prepared and fitter, and they train smarter. It is an amazing fact that many of today's champions are in their mid-to-late thirties. To compete in the toughest sport in the world, at its highest level, at this age, is incredible. I always train to be in the best mental and physical condition possible. There are many benefits of training like a boxer. To get a lean, strong, toned body you have to make a commitment and follow a logical plan. I know that when I finally retire from the ring, I will stay in shape by continuing with the best cross-training routine ever created – the boxer's workout.

The fitness boxing workout is the ultimate cross-training programme that conditions the entire body. This book provides the best of traditional boxing training and combines it with the current approach to elite physical conditioning. It is an exciting and challenging workout that is never boring and is packed full of information on proper technique, conditioning and motivation. After completing the twelve-week programme you may not be ready for a title bout, but you sure will feel like you are.

Ignite your passion for fitness. Box your way to a stronger, leaner, and healthier body and attain the astounding power, agility and endurance of a champion without stepping into the ring.

Sergio 'Maravilla' Martinez

Sergio Martinez was the World Middleweight Champion from 2010 to 2014. He is also the former WBC Super Welterweight Champion. His professional record consists of 51 wins, 3 losses and 2 draws. Sergio was named the 2010 Fighter of the Year by Ring Magazine and at one point in his career he was ranked as one of the top 3 pound-for-pound boxers in the world.

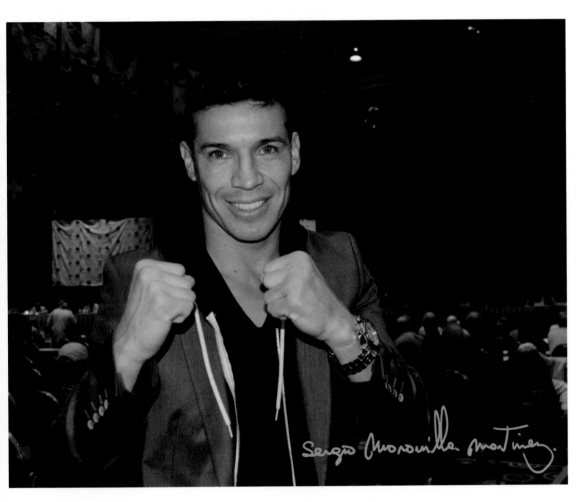

Sergio 'Maravilla' Martinez.

PREFACE

Boxing for fitness has taken the fitness world by storm. That can be good and bad. What is good is that this ancient sport of boxing provides a fantastic workout. The downside is that whenever an activity is adapted for the general public, it can become so watered down that the integrity of the original sport gets lost.

Fitness boxing is not boxercise, cardio-boxing, or plyo-boxing. This book is an introduction to the training of real boxers – what they do to prepare for battle in the ring. Our fitness boxing programme takes the best part of a boxer's training regimen and provides an exhilarating cross-training workout. Guidance is provided for you to learn to train like a boxer, including challenging interval workouts, proper execution of exercises and body awareness, nutritional advice, stretching and recovery.

The science of fitness training has changed dramatically over the years with the advanced knowledge of how the body functions and how it responds to exercise, proper nutrition, strength training, recovery, and relaxation techniques. Boxing training however continues to work with the tried and true principles and training regimens that have not changed for almost one hundred years. Certainly the technology and design of the equipment have evolved and improved, but the heart and soul of the boxer's workout – the heavy bag, speed bag, medicine ball, jump rope, and the committed training schedule – have not changed much. The reason for this is simple. It works.

The programme described here lets you feel your power on the heavy bag, the quick responsiveness resulting from focus mitt training, the heightened foot speed, agility and quickness from jumping rope, the developed musculature from working with the medicine ball, and the resulting improvement of your aerobic capacity from roadwork training. To keep the muscles responsive and healthy, stretching routines are included for each workout, along with nutritional information.

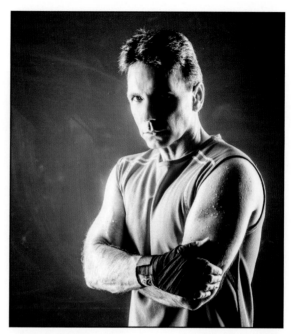

Andy Dumas.

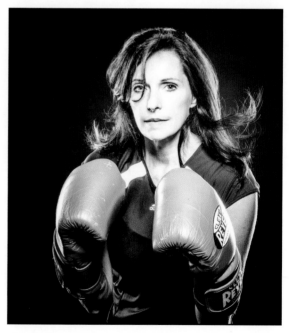

Jamie Dumas.

The training techniques and routines in the book have been inspired by the great boxing champions and coaches of the past and present. Their dedication and passion for the sport reveals the commitment they required on a day-to-day basis to be at their best. These programmes and workout schedules have been developed over a twenty-year period.

Workouts are provided at three training levels of intensity: the basic workout, the contender workout, and finally the champ's workout. All three workouts provide day-to-day progression and give rewarding results. Start at a level that you find challenging, but also one in which suits your current fitness level and lifestyle. You can combine the basic workout with your existing training programme to take your conditioning to another level. The contender and the champ's programmes are designed to get you in the best shape possible in 12 weeks.

The fitness and health benefits of training like a boxer are easily identified in your everyday activities, and you will feel them in your other sporting endeavours. Both beginners and seasoned athletes will benefit from this challenging and exciting training routine. Improved agility, speed, muscle mass, reduction in fat percentage, improved cardiovascular conditioning, core strength, balance, overall health, and stamina – all this can be achieved by committing to our fitness boxing workout.

Andy and Jamie Dumas

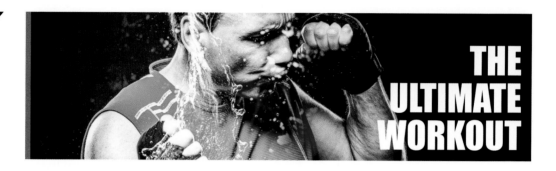

THE ULTIMATE WORKOUT

Fitness boxing replicates the most beneficial elements of a boxer's workout, to maximize results in the shortest amount of time. It is a fun, effective and dynamic routine that includes all aspects of boxing training. This is the place where boxing and fitness meet in perfect balance. As you start to take up fitness boxing, this book will offer you the best of both worlds.

Boxers have to push themselves to the limit when they are in training camp, so they can give maximum effort when they are fighting. If a boxer cuts corners while they are training they will be unable to perform effectively in the ring when it really counts. For the average fitness enthusiast however, the thought of stepping into the ring to face an opponent and take punches is not at the top of their list. Fitness boxing is for those who want to experience the type of training a boxer goes through to get into top shape.

This authentic boxing workout has been developed over years, working with some of the world's best boxers and trainers. Boxing, otherwise known as 'the sweet science', is made palatable for non-boxers by removing sparring from the equation. This eliminates the wear and tear or even the punishment that a boxer may sustain when facing an actual opponent.

WHY IS IT MODELLED ON BOXING?

Why create a workout routine based on a boxer's training regimen? It is simple: because boxers are the best-conditioned athletes in the world. Boxers need the endurance to go the distance, and at the same time require anaerobic conditioning for explosive bursts of speed and power. The key elements of a successful boxer include: superb coordination, muscular

strength, power, foot speed, agility, aerobic endurance and intense anaerobic bursts. At the highest level, boxers must be in superb physical condition and exhibit mental commitment and drive.

A Boxer's Fitness

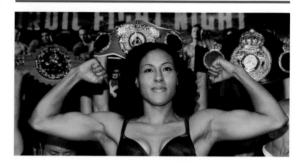

Cecilia Braekhus, Female Welterweight Champion.

'Our training is very special and it covers the entire body. You have to be 100 per cent fit, otherwise you are in trouble. The conditioning is very popular in fitness studios. I know a lot of people who take boxing training just for fitness reasons. There is no better training for your overall fitness.' (Cecilia Braekhus, WBA, WBC, WBO Female Welterweight Champion)

THE PHYSICAL CHARACTERISTICS OF GREAT ATHLETES

The skills and physicality of athletes vary from sport to sport; however there are twelve general physical characteristics all great athletes must possess.

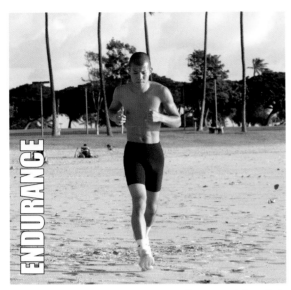

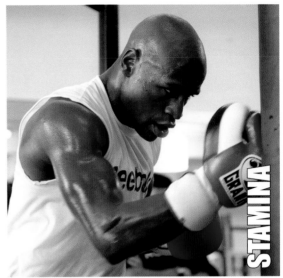

Cardiovascular/Respiratory Endurance: The ability of the body systems to gather, process, and deliver oxygen to the working muscles.

Boxers must have the endurance to perform at an optimal level for the entire fight, and for every round, be it the first round or the last, they must maintain the same level of intensity.

Stamina: The ability of body systems to process, deliver, store, and utilize energy.

Boxers are conditioned to continually move in the ring, using their legs to change direction and manoeuvre into position, and to throw a high volume of effective punches and go the fight distance.

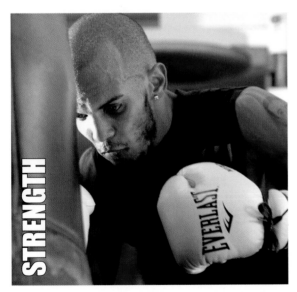

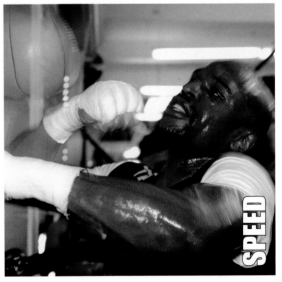

Strength: The ability of a muscular unit, or combination of muscular units, to apply force.

Boxers develop power by delivering forceful punches repeatedly on the heavy bag. The upper body, shoulders, arms, core and leg muscles play an important role in producing strong punches.

Speed: The ability to minimize the time cycle of a repeated movement.

Boxers rapidly throw punch after punch, reducing the amount of time between strikes.

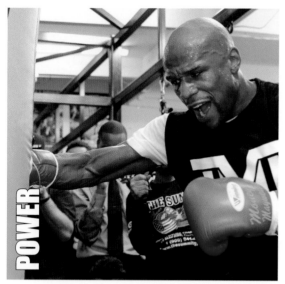

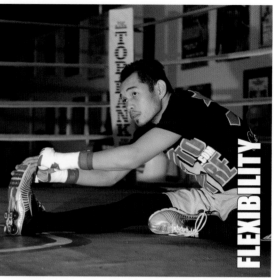

Power: The ability of a muscular unit, or combination of muscular units, to apply maximum force in minimum time.

The combination of strength and speed is essential for boxers; the muscles of the arms, upper body, core, and legs are trained to deliver forceful punches with precise, explosive power.

Flexibility: The ability to maximize the range of motion at a given joint.

Boxers need to be agile, to avoid incoming punches by slipping and ducking; flexible muscles allow for quick movement changes and prevent the risk of muscle tears and injuries to the joint regions.

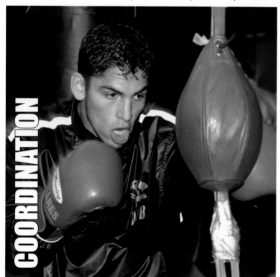

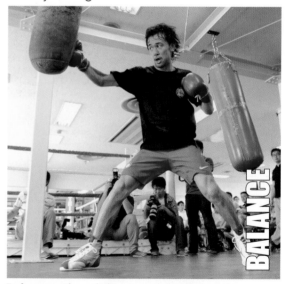

Coordination: The ability to combine several distinct movement patterns into a singular distinct movement.

Boxers develop and execute synchronized punching combinations matched with defensive moves and balanced footwork.

Balance: The ability to control the placement of the body's centre of gravity in relation to its support base.

Boxers are always on the move and develop a strong core and a sense of how to maintain a strong centre of balance; they need to be able to throw punches from awkward angles and to be able to move to maintain their equilibrium after taking punches.

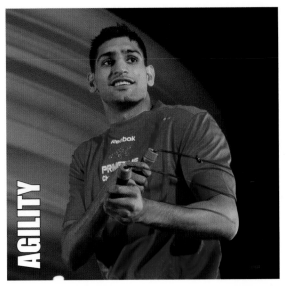

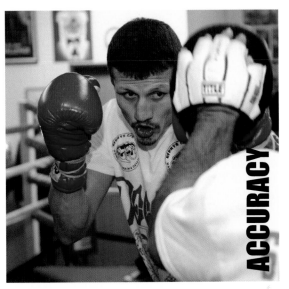

Agility: The ability to minimize transition time from one movement pattern to another.

Boxers are light on their feet, allowing for free-flowing transitions and a variety of punch sequences to be administered.

Accuracy: The ability to control movement in a given direction or at a given intensity.

Boxers train to develop the delivery of the perfect punch or punch sequences to the desired location.

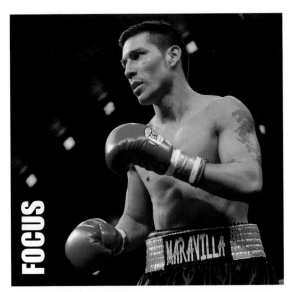

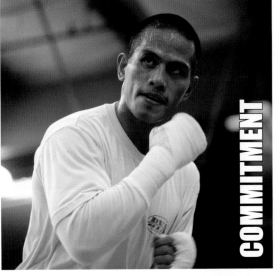

Focus: Concentration on the task at hand, focusing on technique, being in the moment and doing your best.

In no other sport is it more important for an athlete to be 'in the moment'. Good boxers have to be one step ahead of their opponents for the entire bout. They must maintain perfect concentration for every second of every round.

Commitment: Mental commitment and drive, ensuring adherence to a training schedule and the goal at hand.

Boxing champions have the commitment and the intense mental focus required to succeed. Great boxers take pride in the process of developing a strong, lean, healthy body so their every move is executed with perfection.

If you want to achieve the physicality of a great athlete, with quick reflexes, agility, balance, power, and coordination, then you need to train like one. Fitness boxing training mimics the workouts of the best-conditioned athletes in the world. This workout offers variety and is both challenging, stimulating, and never boring. One of the most difficult challenges when pursuing a healthier and a more active lifestyle is being consistent and sticking with the training. The key is to stay inspired and motivated to get the maximum benefit from your commitment.

Motivation to Train

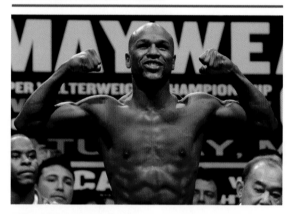

Floyd Mayweather Jr.

'Perhaps the greatest benefit of an entertaining workout is the motivation to exercise when you otherwise might not train.' (Floyd Mayweather Jr, boxing's pound-for-pound champion)

THE TALE OF THE TAPE

The 'tale of the tape' is a boxing term referring to an athlete's prefight measurements, such as height, weight, reach and age. From a fitness point of view this phrase has equally important implications. Everyone has their own unique body type, fast or slow twitch muscle fibres, percentage of fat and musculature, cardiovascular fitness and base starting fitness levels, as well as adaptation rates. Whatever your current level of fitness, it is important to know how your body develops and adapts to training.

Individual Differences

Each individual is unique with distinctive abilities, capabilities and capacities. Age, gender, heredity, past physical history and a current fitness level determine and influence the rate at which everyone improves their level of physical fitness.

The Law of Adaptation

The intention of physical fitness training is to place demands on your body systematically in order to improve the capability, functionality, and capacity to exercise. Your level of physical fitness is indicative of your level of training, and when the correct exercise demands are introduced into the training programme, your fitness level improves. When the exercise demands are not sufficient or cease altogether, then the fitness level plateaus or declines. Once you reach a plateau in your fitness level it is time to change the stresses on the body and introduce new stresses or demands.

The training effect results from the adaptation of the body to the stress of the physical effort required to meet the additional demands. A threshold tension is necessary for improvements to occur. If the stress is not sufficient, then no changes will occur. If the stress is too great, then injury or over-training can occur.

The heart, lungs, muscle, joints, and the immune system all adapt to exercise. The muscles get stronger, the joints become sufficiently lubricated, the bones become stronger and thicker; the heart pumps out a greater volume of blood to the working muscles, and the lungs provide a greater percentage of oxygen to the circulatory system.

Factors involved in the adaptation process include overload, specificity and reversibility, as well as individual differences. All of these will determine the rate and type of physical gain you will obtain.

Overload Principle

The stress or demands of an action or activity must be greater than what the body is accustomed to in order for an overload to take place. The additional required exertion places elevated demands on the varying systems of the body. Just by starting a different training programme, new demands or overloads are placed on the body and fitness level improvements can be acknowledged quickly.

When your body adapts to the training overload placed upon it, accommodation will occur. Accommodation is when there is no longer any additional progress in your fitness level. It is the result of the body successfully adapting to the training stimuli and is often referred to as reaching a plateau.

When a fitness level plateau has been reached and limited improvement in your fitness level is recognized, a new overload must be added to your training programme. The way to avoid or overcome a fitness level plateau and progressively improve is to provide sufficient variety in your training regimen. Ways to provide variety in your training are to modify the rest time between the exercises, change the speed or the rate at which the exercise is executed, change the number of sets and/or repetitions of an exercise, change the exercise or the order in which you perform the exercise, and increase the load or demand. Variety in the types of exercise and methods of execution are the keys to providing an ongoing overload to the body.

Exercise choices and time allotments need to be considered, and rest intervals are very important to maximize the overload tensions. With adequate rest and sufficient recovery time, the body will get stronger and fitness levels will improve. For those who are new to fitness training, it will take the body a few months to adapt to the new demands of the activity and variety is not as imperative.

Specificity

The body adapts specifically to the type of stress and demands that are placed upon it and therefore the type of adaptation results from the actual training regimen. A good training programme places stress on the muscles that are required to perform a specific movement and also include muscle movements that are as close as possible to the activity that you want to improve.

There are a number of types of specificity such as: speed of a muscle contraction, the sequence of a movement, the speed of a movement, specific motor patterns and synchronicity, and the power behind the movement. A variety of exercises are included in the training schedule to provide a sufficient overload for continued athletic progress giving an effective total body workout.

Reversibility or Un-Adaptation

If you do not exercise and do not place specific demands or an overload on the body, your fitness level not only plateaus, but it will reverse to a lower level. When a muscle is not used or has been immobilized, atrophy will occur. This means the strength and the mass of the muscle will decrease. The joints lose their lubrication and become dry, the bones become brittle, the heart rate increases and less oxygen is delivered to the working muscles. You become de-conditioned.

Benefits of Exercise

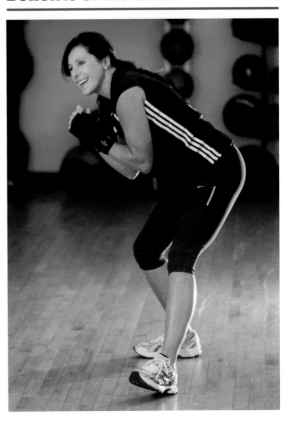

The physical and psychological benefits of exercising are numerous, including weight control and the reduction of such diseases as cardiovascular disease, type 2 diabetes, and some cancers. Staying active and following an exercise programme will increase bone density as well as diminish joint pain. Muscle strength is improved and the ageing process is slowed down. Exercising elevates self-esteem and has a positive effect on mental health.

TRAINING INTENSITIES

To obtain the greatest return from your workout, train with intensity, commitment and consistency. Get to know yourself and how hard to push when training. There will be days when your body will respond as you want it to, and there will be days when you will feel sluggish and slow.

Rate of Perceived Exertion (RPE)

How hard do you have to work to achieve the fitness level you want? One of the more simple ways to measure and monitor how hard you are working or your 'exercising intensity' is to use a Rate of Perceived Exertion scale: 0–10.

This scale is based on a 0–10 level chart rating how you feel when physically exerting yourself. While you are sitting in a chair at rest the exertion rating is zero. When you move your arms while sitting in a chair the rating is 1. Warming up before exercising helps to increase the blood flow to your muscles and the rating is 2–3. Walking at a moderate pace is a rating of 3. When it is very difficult to continue the activity for more than a minute, like sprints or speed work, the rating is 9–10.

Regardless of your current fitness level or the type of training you are performing, using RPE to gauge your exercise intensity is effective and helpful. Basically your effort, fatigue or discomfort experienced during either cardio activities or resistance training can be correlated to the RPE scale. The scale typically shows a linear relationship of how hard your heart is working and the quantity of oxygen being consumed with the amount of exertion you believe you are generating.

Using the scale is simple and uncomplicated, no equipment is required, and you do not have to stop the activity to get a reading. It is easy to continually monitor how you feel and therefore how hard you are working whether you are running, jumping rope, hitting the bag or performing focus mitt drills. Adjust your workout intensity level up or down to correspond to the scale, and then train at this desired rate.

Perceived exertion accounts for increases and decreases in the heart rate, other physiological changes in the body, and also allows for psychological factors that may influence your training capabilities. Learn to listen to your body and be aware of how you are feeling.

By choosing a workout with a wide variety of fitness training options, setting realistic goals for yourself, making physical activity a priority in your everyday life and adopting a healthy diet, you can acquire superior overall physical conditioning and well-being. Fitness boxing provides an exhilarating and enjoyable workout to help you achieve maximum results in the most efficient way possible, achieving improvements in muscular strength and endurance, cardiovascular and respiratory endurance, flexibility and body composition.

RPE SCALE

0-1	No exertion. Sitting in a chair and relaxed.
2-3	Light exertion. Warm-up exercises, stretching, cooling down. Your muscles are starting to warm up.
4-5	Medium exertion. Heart rate increases slightly, breathing slightly faster, and your body is getting warmer.
6-7	Moderate exertion. Your breathing increases and you will start to sweat. Talking will become an effort.
8-9	Hard exertion. Your breathing becomes more laboured and it is difficult to talk.
10	Hardest exertion. You have difficulty keeping this pace for more than 1 minute – then this is your limit. You will be unable to speak.

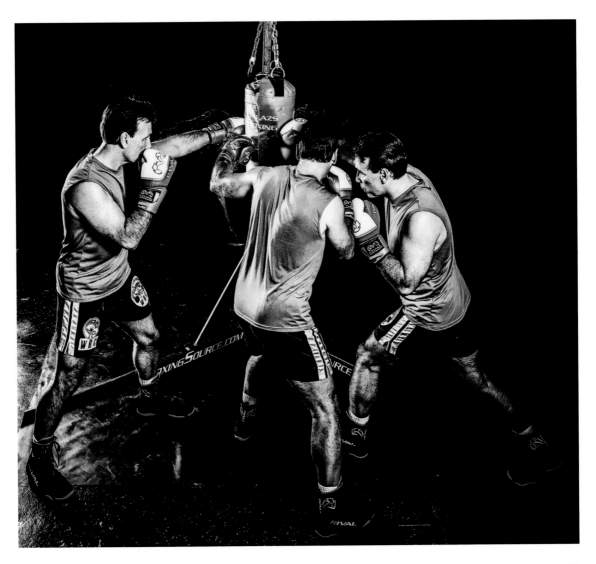

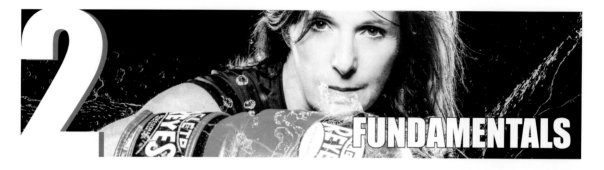

To build a strong foundation for an effective fitness boxing workout, the basic fundamentals must be practised properly. Your fitness level and skills will progress naturally if you take the time to master the fundamentals. When developing new skills, aim to make them a habit. A habit is a conditioned reflex that is the result of repetitive movements. The goal is to practise the fundamental skills until they become 'good' habits.

Think about it...

'I love the technical part of training, that to me is the most fascinating. It's a combination of so many things. How you coordinate your footwork with your defence and offense, or the combination of balance and strength. That is really fascinating to me. You always keep learning, you are never done!' (Cecilia Braekhus, Female World Welterweight Champion)

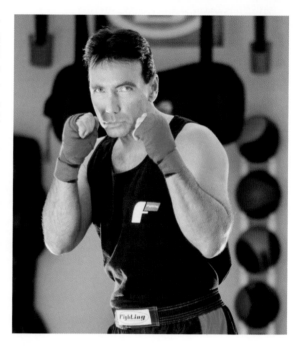

Traditional boxing stance.

THE TRADITIONAL BOXING STANCE

All moves in boxing originate from a balanced boxing stance. It is the foundation of smooth, steady movement that facilitates the delivery of effective punch combinations. It is essential that you develop a boxing stance that provides stability and allows you to move easily.

Determining Your Correct Stance

If your dominant hand is your right hand, adopt a 'classic' or 'orthodox' stance. The left shoulder and the left foot are forward, allowing for the easy execution of the left jab. Developing a solid, left jab will allow you to set up power punches such as the straight right. If your dominant hand is your left hand, then the right shoulder and right foot are forward, and you will utilize a right jab. This is referred to as 'southpaw stance'.

Throughout this book, all moves and combinations will be described from the classic/orthodox stance.

Foot Placement

Proper foot placement is one of the most important elements for an effective boxing stance. If your foot placement is not correct

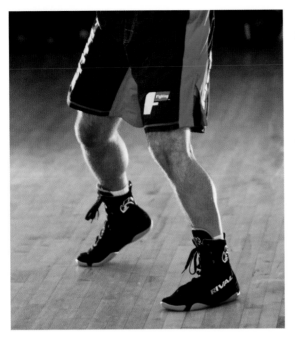

Foot placement.

The foot position and the three-quarter stance should feel balanced and allow easy movement in all directions. Your knees should be slightly bent allowing for better mobility, power and balanced movement. Make sure not to bend your knees too much as this will result in clumsy and sluggish movement.

The Body

Your body position is angled and slightly sideways providing the smallest target area possible. Your front shoulder, front hip and forward foot line up. Keep your abdominals firm and your shoulders slightly rounded, forward and relaxed. Focus on the centre of your body and start all your movements from deep within your core. The power of your punch is generated from a strong, centred core.

The Arms and Shoulders

Hold your arms close to the sides of the body by the ribcage, with your shoulders relaxed and slightly rounded. The elbows are bent and pointing down and in, thereby protecting your ribcage and solar plexus. Keep both hands up by your face. Boxers are constantly adjusting the position of their arms in order to defend against body shots and headshots from their opponents.

The Hands and Fists

On-guard position

Your fists stay up high to protect your face and chin. Close your fingers together to make a loose fist, with your thumb folding to the outside of the fingers. Ensure you do not clench your fist too tightly. Turn your fists inward slightly and keep your wrists strong and straight. The orthodox boxer holds the right fist slightly higher, very close to the chin, while the left fist is held just above the top of the left shoulder. It is from this position that all punches are executed (reverse for southpaws).

Your fists are always in the on-guard position unless you are throwing a punch. Quickly bring your fist directly back to protect your head again after throwing a punch.

you will be unable to move effectively and efficiently when shadow boxing, working the heavy bags or working on the focus mitts. Your front (lead) foot should point toward your imaginary opponent. (The heavy bag and your partner on the focus mitts are considered your 'opponent'.)

It is essential to start with a solid base to execute all moves. Stand with your feet shoulder width apart or slightly wider. Step backward with your right foot. The back or trail foot is behind and slightly off to the side of your front foot and never directly behind your front lead foot. This is the starting foot position for an orthodox (right-hand dominant) boxer.

Equally distribute your body weight approximately 50/50 between the front and back foot. Too much weight on your front foot makes it difficult to move and step away quickly after you have thrown a punch. It also reduces the ability to pivot on the trail foot and decreases the power behind your straight right. Centre your body weight through the balls of your feet, with the heel of the back foot slightly raised. The raised back heel assists you in moving and responding quickly, and allows for an easy foot pivot when throwing power punches.

The Head

Always keep your eyes in the direction of the target (the various punching bags or focus mitts). Your chin stays tucked in toward your chest and your head slightly forward and down. Your right fist and left shoulder provide protection for the chin.

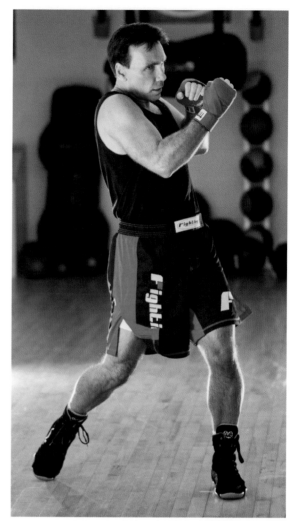

Focus on proper execution of your punches.

Key Points: Boxing Stance

- Keep your legs and feet in a balanced stance ready to move.
- Ensure your body weight is equally centred through the balls of your feet.
- Your front/lead foot points in the direction of your target.
- The toe of the trail foot is pointing out slightly to the side.
- Your back/trail foot is shoulder-width (or more) behind and slightly out to the side of your lead foot, and not directly behind your lead foot.
- Keep your body relaxed, in particular the neck and shoulder muscles, for easier execution of the punches.
- Keeping your knees slightly bent and staying on the balls of your feet will allow you to move quickly and efficiently from one position to the next.
- Your front shoulder, hip and foot are aligned and your body angles toward the target.
- Your arms are held close to the sides of the body with your elbows positioned by the rib cage.
- Close your fingers in a loose fist, with your thumb resting over the top of the fingers.
- Your fists turn in slightly and are held high in the on-guard position.
- Keep your core muscles held tight.

The correct execution of each single punch must be duplicated over and over in order to improve your skill. Develop a multitude of smooth and technically correct single punches before working on punch combinations. Practise with purpose and stay focused on throwing one effective punch at a time. Your muscles need to be trained to react quickly and simultaneously to produce effective punches.

The basic punches that need to be mastered are the jab, straight right, hooks, and uppercuts. Focus on proper execution of your individual punches and then they will become an instantaneous movement or habit.

The Left Jab

A fast, effective jab is a boxer's number one weapon. The main purpose of the jab is to keep your opponent at a safe distance, distracted and off-guard. It sets up more dangerous punches such as the straight right and hooks. The jab should be thrown with speed and accuracy. In a boxing match the jab is the most frequently thrown punch in your arsenal, (about 65–70 per cent of the total punches thrown). Developing an effective jab will accomplish many things; it can be thrown accurately from multiple angles while you are moving, and can be utilized as both an offensive and defensive weapon. During any given round, whether shadow boxing or on the heavy bag, jabs should be thrown almost continually.

For a boxer standing in the traditional or orthodox stance, the left jab starts with your palm facing you and your hand in a relaxed fist. Your left arm snaps away from your body in a straight line toward the target. As your arm extends forward, your fist rotates and your palm faces down at point of impact. Fully extend your arm without any hyperextension at your elbow. Allow your shoulder to follow through to protect your chin. When you launch the jab do not rotate your fist too early. Allow the rotation to flow from the movement that starts from your shoulder, extends through your elbow and then to your fist. Keep your elbow moving forward and by the side of your body, as the very common mistake of raising the elbow out to the side makes the punch weak, ineffective and telegraphs the punch.

After striking your target, bring your left arm back to the on-guard position quickly and along the same path of the delivery. Protect your ribs by keeping your elbows close to the sides of your body. Keep your right hand by your face when throwing the left jab.

Jabs can be thrown to an opponent's head or body. When throwing punches to the body, bend your knees to lower the position of your punch, rather than dropping your hands. This can be practised when shadowboxing or training on the heavy bag.

Initially there should be very little movement from your body as you practise your jab. Once the effectiveness of your punch improves increase your punch power by moving forward slightly as you launch your jab. To accomplish this, push off the ball of your back foot slightly and slide your front foot forward at the same time as you throw the punch. Your foot movement must be synchronized with your punch. Always execute your jab from a well-balanced position and breathe naturally exhaling as you launch your punch. Get in the habit of snapping your jabs. Throw them often and with speed.

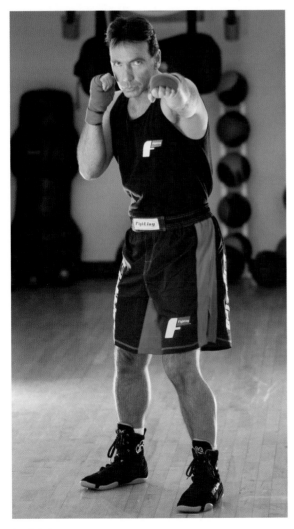

Left jab.

> ## Key Points: Left Jab
> - Avoid the 'chicken wing' effect (this is when your elbow leaves the side of the body creating a sloppy and ineffective punch). Keep your elbow moving straight forward as you execute your jab and do not lift it out sideways.
> - Winding-up or pulling back the fist is another common mistake. Practise in front of a mirror to make sure you are throwing your jab straight out and returning it straight back to the on-guard position.
> - Rotate your fist during the last third of the punch so your palm is facing down on impact. Focus on fully extending your arm and rotating your fist.
> - Throw plenty of fast, snappy, crisp jabs.

The Straight Right

The straight right is a power punch executed from the orthodox boxing stance. It is similar to throwing a jab with your powerful dominant hand instead of the lead hand. Starting in the on-guard stance, your right hand is thrown from the chin as your rear shoulder thrusts forward. The fist travels in a straight line toward the target and rotates during the last third of the punch with your palm facing down.

The straight right takes more time and more energy to execute than the jab. Power is generated off your trail foot and the punch travels straight forward to the target. Remember to tighten your core muscles to maintain correct alignment and a strong centre of balance. Stay on the balls of your feet and in the three-quarter stance with your right hip rotating forward. The simultaneous rotation of the right hip and right shoulder along with the push-off of the ball of your rear foot, combine to produce a powerful straight right.

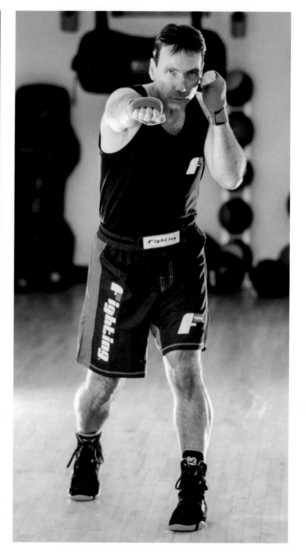

Straight right.

As with the jab, ensure that you do not pull the arm or lift your rear elbow before throwing the punch. Keep your lead hand in front of the face to protect your chin. Finish the punch with your hips square to the target, your chin down and both eyes on the target. Swiftly return to the on-guard position as you prepare to throw your next punch. More muscles are engaged and more energy is required when throwing straight rights.

The straight right is often referred to as the right-cross. The intent of the right-cross is the same as the straight right with a slight variation in the execution. The right-cross is launched when an opponent has thrown a left jab and your straight right power punch must be thrown with a slight arc over and across the left jab, unlike the straight right which is thrown in a straight line to the target.

Key Points: Straight Right

- Make sure your shoulders and hips move together and your body weight is transferring from your back foot to your front foot when the punch is launched.
- Do not lift your rear elbow. Execute the punch in a straight line to the target.
- Think of the punch as a synchronized body movement, with your knees slightly bent for easy rotation of your torso, shoulders and hip regions.
- Keep up on the ball of your rear foot as you launch the punch.
- Keep the lead (jab) fist in the on-guard position. Do not let it drop as you execute the straight right.

Hooks

The hook is a short-range, semi-circular punch most often thrown with your lead hand. These short, damaging punches are set up with jabs or straight-rights. The power of the hook does not come from the arm swing alone. The strength and velocity of this punch comes from the synchronization of the body pivoting while rotating through the hips and pressing through the feet. In order for hooks to be effective, they must to be thrown at close range. It is not a wild punch, but rather a punch thrown with precision and control.

The Left Hook

When this compact punch is properly executed at close range, it is often outside your opponent's range of vision and offers the element of surprise.

With your hands in the on-guard position and your core muscles held tight, keep your knees slightly bent and your body weight centred through both of your legs. As you launch the punch, your left elbow lifts away from the rib cage and the underside of your arm is parallel to the floor. The elbow is kept at a 90-degree angle throughout the delivery.

Your shoulders and hips rotate clockwise and your lead foot pivots inward on the ball of your foot. Your wrist remains strong and your thumb points up, allowing your knuckles to make solid contact. Quickly return your left

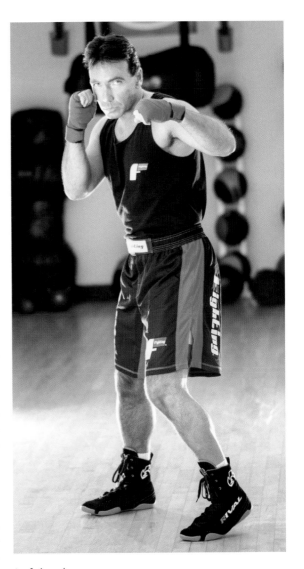

Left hook.

elbow to the side of the body with your left fist up to protect the chin.

One advantage of an effective left hook is the short distance it travels to reach the target. The left hook moves about one-third of the distance of the straight right, making it a very deceptive punch. The hook can be delivered to the body or the head. By bending your knees your body is lowered and puts you in the ideal position to launch a hook to the body.

The Right Hook

For an orthodox boxer, the right hook comes from your dominant rear hand. It has a greater distance to travel to make contact. It is not utilized as much as the left hook in a boxing match since the opponent can easily detect the wide-hooking motion coming off the back foot. Your body moves the same way as when you throw a straight right, but your right arm swings in a tight circular motion. You must step in closer to your target, as your arm is not extended fully. A flurry of short left and right hooks to the body can be thrown at close range when working the heavy bag.

Key Points: Hooks

- Move your arm and upper body as one unit and pivot on the ball of your left (front) foot when throwing a left hook, and on the ball of your right (rear) foot when throwing the right hook.
- Move in and launch your punch when you are close to the target. A common mistake is to launch the punch when you are too far away.
- Do not throw big, looping hooks. Throw short, compact hooks.
- Keep your elbow bent at 90 degrees and at shoulder level.

Pivot on the ball of your rear foot, quickly rotating your arm, shoulder, body, and hips in one movement in a counter-clockwise direction. After the punch is thrown, quickly return to the on-guard position, fists up by your chin and elbows protecting your body.

Uppercut

Uppercuts are powerful, close-range punches and can be thrown by either the left or the right hand. The punch travels in an upward arc motion toward the target. Like the hook, this punch is considered an inside punch and you must be close to the target. Uppercuts can be delivered to your opponent's body or the chin.

Right Uppercut

To launch the right uppercut, begin in the orthodox stance keeping your rear knee relaxed with a slight bend. Your right shoulder lowers to the right side of the body and the left fist stays high by your chin and head for protection. From this semi-crouching position, rotate your hips forward, throwing your fist upward in a rising arc toward the target. Your arm remains bent at the elbow, your wrist stays strong, and your right shoulder follows through with the rotating hips. Use the power of your legs by pushing up quickly through your knees. Upon impact, square your hips front and keep your elbows bent at a right angle. All of this occurs simultaneously in one smooth movement. Return to the on-guard position as quickly as possible, ready for the next move.

Left Uppercut

The left uppercut is thrown by positioning your body in a semi-crouching position to the left side, with your left shoulder lowered and your body weight transferring to the ball of your left foot upon delivery of the punch. Keep the punch motion tight, using an upward driving force from your hips and legs to increase the power of the punch on impact. An uppercut thrown from a long range will lose some of its power because the arm is no longer sufficiently bent at the elbow and the total body's force will not be transferred in the upward movement. Learn to set up your uppercuts with

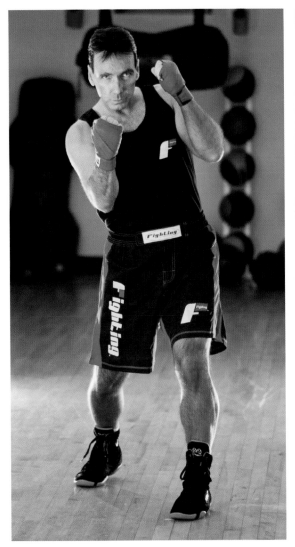

Right uppercut.

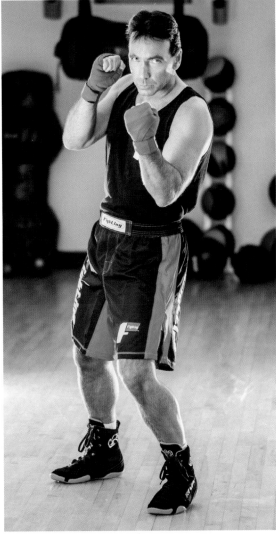

Left uppercut.

Key Points: Uppercuts

- Do not wind up or take your arm back before you throw this punch.
  Not only is this ineffective, but this loopy punch can be injurious to your shoulder.
- Use the power and strength behind your body by transferring your weight foward and in the direction of your punch.
- Drive off the balls of your feet in order to execute the uppercut. Do not lean backward onto your heel. Keep your balance centred, with your core muscles held tight.
- At the time of delivery and follow through, your elbow remains bent at a 90-degree angle for the most impact.

Hybrid Punches

There are dozens of different ways to throw each punch, and depending on your body position, the timing of the punch execution, your body build and individual idiosyncrasies, some of the punches you throw will be of a hybrid nature.

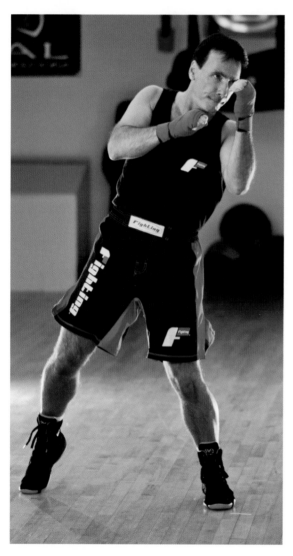

Hybrid punch.

Inventing Your Own Punch

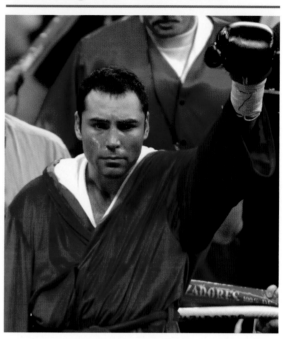

'I use my left hand to throw a punch that I call my 45 because it comes at a 45-degree angle, somewhere between a hook and an uppercut. It has to do with the angle of my arm and from that unique position, it is an effective and powerful punch.' (Oscar De La Hoya)

De La Hoya's 45 was indeed a unique punch. It was not quite a hook, it was not quite an uppercut, but rather it was a hybrid of the two. Master the basic punches and fundamentals first and then you can develop your own unique style of punching.

Counterpunching

A counterpunch is a punch that you launch immediately after a punch has been thrown at you. This counter-attack takes advantage of your opponent not being in the protective on-guard position. Visualize an opponent throwing a punch, then slip or duck and come back with creative counterpunches of your own. This skill will be developed further in the focus mitt chapter. An example of one of the greatest counterpunchers in boxing history is Floyd Mayweather Jr (see internet fight-footage of his incredible counterpunching ability and the resulting victories).

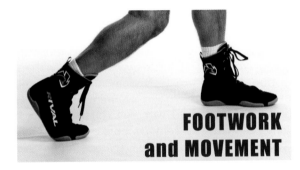

FOOTWORK and MOVEMENT

Muhammad Ali took imaginative footwork and ingenious movement in the ring to a balletic art form. His balance, rhythm and ability to change direction looked almost effortless. High quality footwork is important in many sports such as soccer and tennis, but in no other sport is it more important than in boxing.

Skilful footwork can get a boxer out of dangerous situations and provide counterpunching opportunities. Developing smooth and balanced footwork is also essential for an effective fitness boxing workout. Footwork should be calculated and have a purpose. Use your legs and feet to get you into and out of punching range. Stay relaxed and in control. Maintain your balance and stay on the balls of your feet. This will allow you to move smoothly across the floor.

Feet First
Moving Forward
Starting from the balanced boxing stance, push off the ball of your trail foot as you move your front or lead foot forward. Remember to stay light on your feet and land on the ball of your front foot. The purpose of the forward movement is to get you into range to land punches, such as the jab or straight right. Finding your range and stride distance to set up your perfect punch will take practice.

Moving Backward
Retreating movements are necessary to avoid an opponent's punches. To move backward push off your front foot as the trail foot moves back. The purpose of moving backward is to reset and plan your next move. This may involve punching or moving again in another direction.

Moving Left
This movement is not a lunge and should be kept compact. Keep your feet shoulder-width apart in order to maintain your balance. To move left, push off your rear (right) foot as your front (left) foot moves to the left. When moving to the left ensure that you are keeping your ¾ stance facing the target and you are not standing square to the target.

Key Points: Footwork

- Do not try to cover ground too quickly by lunging or taking huge steps. This will put you off balance and in an awkward position.
- Do not cross your feet to change direction.
- Come back to the balanced on-guard position quickly, keeping your front foot and shoulder in the direction of the target.
- When moving forward, push off the ball of your trail foot at the same time as you move your front foot forward.
- When moving backward, push off your front foot as your trail foot moves back.
- When moving to the left, push off your rear (right) foot as your front (left) foot moves to the left.
- When moving to the right, push off your front (left) foot as you move your rear (right) foot to the right.

Moving Right

When moving to the right, push off your front (left) foot as you move your rear (right) foot to the right. Try to move your feet at the same time. Always stay in the orthodox boxing stance when moving.

General Foot Movement

Think in terms of 'pushing off' instead of 'stepping'. Both feet move almost simultaneously with your lead foot moving a split second first. If you take a large step with the lead foot first, your weight will be placed on the heel instead of the ball of the lead foot, making it difficult to change directions quickly. Pushing off keeps you on the balls of your feet and allows you to move quickly and pivot easily.

Bouncing Rhythm

Bouncing rhythm, also called boxer's rhythm or boxer's bounce, refers to a style of boxing movement that involves energetic bouncing and footwork similar to jumping rope. It is generally a forward and backward movement that is balanced and subtle. The punches are timed with the bounce motion. This style of footwork provides cardio-conditioning, burns more calories and keeps you light on your feet.

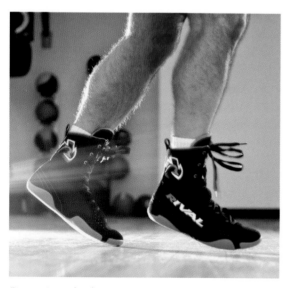

Bouncing rhythm.

Watch old fight footage of Muhammad Ali or Sugar Ray Leonard. Notice how their rhythmic bouncing styles of constantly moving forward, backward, and side-to-side would confuse their opponents and create openings to land their own punches. Their foot movement was smooth and perfectly timed with the release of their punches. A more recent example of a champion who incorporates this lively style of fighting is Sergio Martinez. His entire offence is based on his rhythmic footwork and constant movement around the ring and requires incredible conditioning to keep this up over twelve rounds.

To execute a bouncing rhythm, start in your balanced boxing stance with your knees relaxed. Push off the balls of your feet, similar to jumping rope, and spring slightly off the floor forward, backward, and side-to-side. You must stay on the balls of your feet while moving and your heels should not touch the ground. To move forward push off the ball of your rear foot and land on the ball of your front foot. To move backward, push off the ball of your rear foot and land on the ball of your front foot. This light and 'springy' motion is very subtle and your feet lift just a few centimetres off the ground. You must briefly stop the bouncing motion in order to set your feet and throw your punches before returning to the bouncing rhythm. Bounce, then set your feet, punch, and repeat.

Unnecessarily bouncing back and forth wastes energy and serves no purpose. Each foot pattern should be calculated to put you in position to strike your opponent or avoid counterpunches from your opponent. Practise this style of moving in 20- or 30-second spurts while shadowboxing or hitting the heavy bag. Focus on moving easily in any direction while staying balanced.

SHADOW BOXING

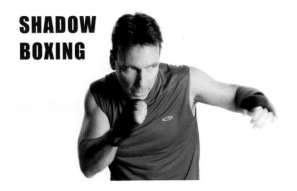

Shadowboxing allows you to incorporate all elements of boxing movement. It is performed without a bag or a partner. The punches, footwork and defensive moves are all combined to create a smooth routine.

Perform shadowboxing at the beginning of any fitness boxing training session. It is not only a great way to warm up the muscles of the body, but it also prepares you mentally for the workout ahead, and allows you to work on proper execution of the punches and foot movements. Shadowboxing is an extremely important facet of fitness boxing training, and boxers will often fill up their spare time between rounds of bag work and skipping with short bursts of shadowboxing.

Your emphasis should be on free flowing body movement and footwork. Your movements, punches and foot patterns should follow a logical sequence and leave you in a balanced position. Remember to move and punch, making use of whatever floor space is available. Shadowboxing is also a great time to practise new combinations and review basic fundamentals. Your job is to visualize an opponent in front of you and perform the necessary moves, be it attacking or defending. Shadowboxing puts you in the ring with your opponent.

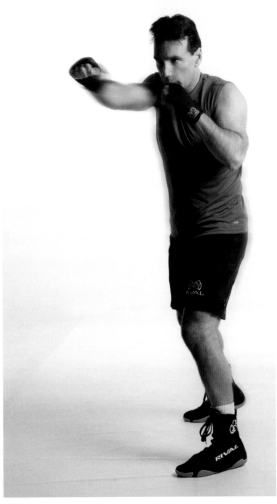

Shadowbox with a virtual opponent.

Throw some jabs as you move into position to strike your imaginary opponent and then move around. Review the technicalities of your jab ensuring the movement is smooth and accurate. Continue to move in multiple directions throwing crisp jabs.

Shadowboxing Basics

Start by practising your footwork moving in a variety of directions, remembering to stay light on your feet and never crossing your legs. Always keep your hands in the on-guard position when you are shadowboxing.

One-two Combo

As you become more comfortable with the single punches start to put two and three punch combinations together. Throw a jab, followed by a straight right. This is the classic one-two combination. Focus on throwing the combination smoothly and always returning promptly to the on-guard position. This is a combination that you will return to over and over and is the starting point for many multiple punch combinations.

Get creative and add variety to your punch combinations. Double up on your punches. Throw two fast jabs or two hooks consecutively. Visualize throwing punches to your opponent's body by bending your knees and lowering your body position. Throw a quick left jab or a one-two combination to the body. Now rise up quickly and throw some punches in the direction of the head.

Punch Sequencing

Boxing coaches often work with simple number sequences to designate specific punch combinations. (More detail will be given on number sequencing and punch combinations in the focus mitt chapter.) It is however, a good time to start to practise with the number sequencing while you are shadowboxing. The jab is the most important punch and is always designated as 'one'. The straight right usually follows the jab and is designated as 'two'. The left hook is identified as 'three' and the right uppercut is known as 'four'.

As you execute a single punch, the movement should leave you in the proper position to deliver your next punch. If the first move puts you off balance slightly, the next move should put you back on balance. An example of a combination that demonstrates the desired smooth transitional movements is a 'one–two–three' combination: a left jab, followed by a straight right and finishing with a left hook. Start this combination by throwing a quick left jab (1). Next your hips rotate as you pivot on your trail foot and a straight right is launched (2). This should now you leave you in position to throw a left hook (3). As you deliver the left hook, bring your hand back into the on-guard position, ready for your next punch. This simple three-punch combination teaches you to transfer your weight while pivoting on the balls of your feet and staying balanced. Practise this three-punch combination until you are proficient at it and then add on more punches.

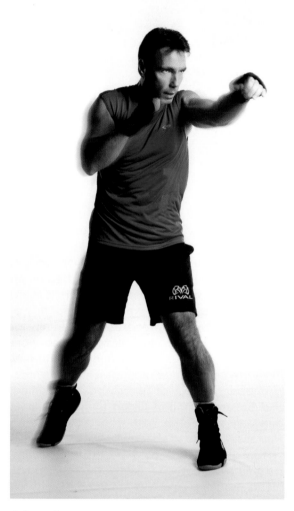

Jab and move.

Keep your combinations simple at first as you decide what punches you want to throw and the desired location of your punch. If you are having trouble with your punch combinations, slow down your punches slightly, throw fewer punches and focus on proper form. There is no benefit to throwing sloppy punches. Ensure you are executing all moves correctly to develop positive muscle memory. Punching speed and punching power will come later.

Key Points: Shadowboxing

- Protect your chin.
- Bring your hands back to the on-guard position after every punch sequence.
- Use the floor space, never standing in one place.
- Stay on balance, timing your foot work with your punches.

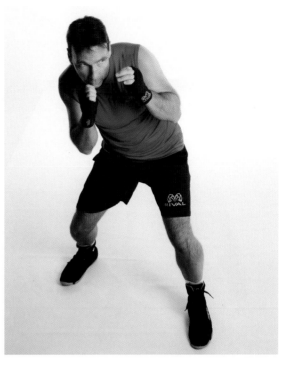

Slip right.

DEFENSIVE MOVES

Mastering defensive moves is essential to be a successful boxer. For fitness boxing, incorporating slips, ducks and feints adds an element of realism to your shadowboxing training. Core and leg muscles are also required to perform these moves, making shadowboxing an effective workout.

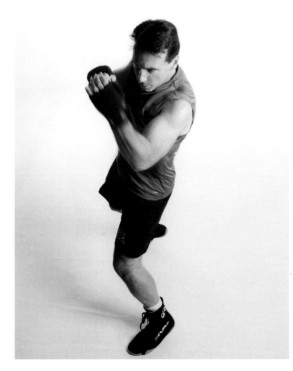

Throw smooth combinations.

Slips

One way boxers avoid getting hit by punches is to 'slip' out of the way. Slipping utilizes a side-to-side motion of your head and upper body allowing evasion of an oncoming punch. Learning to slip effectively also allows boxers to stay in range to throw counterpunches of their own.

To slip punches, start with your hands up in the on-guard position and your body weight slightly forward, then dip to the right or the left and immediately return to your original stance. Always keep your target in view. Although it is mostly an upper body move, the legs play an important role in slipping. Keep your knees bent and think of your legs as shock absorbers assisting in moving you quickly from side to side. Stay on the balls of your feet and do not lean back on your heels.

Incorporating slipping moves in between your punch combinations provides additional fitness benefits such as the use of your core muscles and the expenditure of more calories.

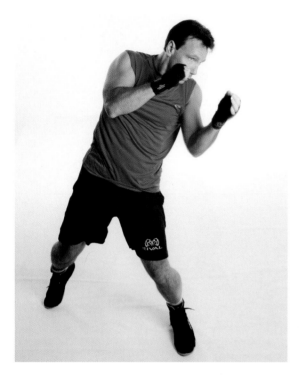

Slip left.

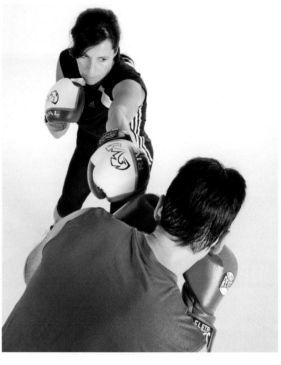

Visualize slipping a left jab.

Slip a Left Jab

Visualize a left jab coming from your opponent, then dip to the right by shifting your body to the right. Your right knee will bend slightly.

Slip a Straight Right

Visualize a straight right coming from your opponent, then dip to the left by shifting your body to the left. Your left knee will bend slightly.

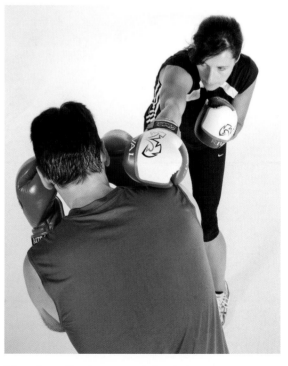

Visualize slipping a straight right.

Key Points: Slips

- Make sure you do not over-slip by shifting your weight too much to one side. Stay centred over your feet.
- Keep your hands close to your chin in the on-guard protective position when slipping.

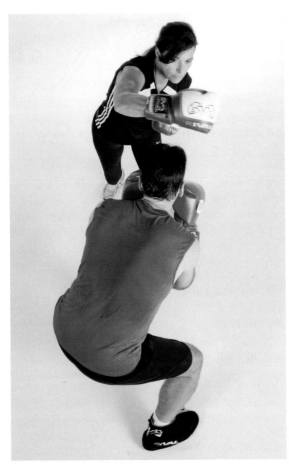

> ### Key Points: Ducking
> - Bend your knees to lower the body. Do not bend at your waist.
> - Stay on the balls of your feet and use your legs.
> - Keep ducks quick and tight, and do not bend too low.

Feints

A feint is a calculated action or movement with the intent to deceive your opponent. By making your opponent think you are going to do one thing but then doing another, you can create opportunities to land punches. You can use shoulder and arm feints to confuse your opponent. Pretend to punch, but do not throw the punch. You can also use your feet to test your opponent's reaction by pretending to move in one direction, then move in another direction. Pretend to direct the punch to one region of the body and then go to a different part of the body. For example, start by aiming your punch at the body, but quickly redirect the punch to the head. Feints should be subtle and not obvious.

Visualize ducking under a right hook.

Ducking

Another defensive method boxers use to avoid getting hit is called 'ducking'. Ducking, also known as 'bobbing and weaving', is utilized against big powerful inside punches like hooks.

Starting in the balanced boxing stance, keep your back straight and bend both knees to 'drop' or lower your body in one quick motion. The motion is very similar to performing a quick squat. This is generally a small downward movement, not going any lower than 90 degrees at the knees. The idea is to duck just enough for the oncoming punch to safely go over the top of your head. Always return to your on-guard position as quickly as possible.

Incorporating ducking moves into your punching routine will give you more of a total body workout, working the core muscles, gluteus, hamstrings and quadriceps.

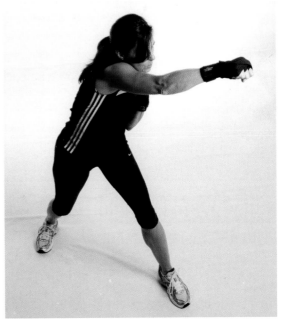

Feint with a left jab and throw a straight right.

Shoulder Feint

Jerk your left shoulder forward as though you are going to throw a jab, but throw a straight right instead.

Foot Feint

Half step with your front foot, looking like you are moving left, then step back circling to the right and throw a left jab.

Punch Feint

Swiftly move just your right hand forward as if you are going to throw a straight right and then come back with a left hook.

Body Punch Feint

Bend your knees and drop down low in a position to throw a punch to the body. Quickly rise up and throw a punch to the head.

Adding feints to your punching routine while shadowboxing, working the target mitts and hitting the heavy bags makes for a more realistic boxing experience. Remember you are trying to replicate a real fighting scenario. If you want to watch a master at feinting, view fight-footage of Roberto Duran, 'the Hands of Stone'.

Key Points: Feints

- Keep the movement subtle. Do not over-exaggerate your feints.
- Practise in front of a mirror to sharpen this skill and to ensure the movement is realistic.
- Return your fists to the on-guard position quickly so that you are in the correct position to execute your punch.

SHADOWBOXING PRACTICE

With a Virtual Opponent

Have a mental image of your opponent and what you want to achieve. Try to find a comfortable rhythm as you punch and move around, matching the footwork and the punches together. Throw a multitude of punches working at a quick pace. Always keep moving, using lateral movement and staying on your toes. Make use of imagery to slip and duck the punches of your 'opponent'.

Shadowboxing at a fast pace for 3-minute rounds will prepare your body for working on the focus mitts and on the heavy bag. Work hard enough so that you feel slightly out of breath, and ready and eager for more. Utilize the 1-minute rest in between rounds to imagine new defensive scenarios and plan creative punch combinations. Always have a purpose when you shadowbox, and vary the selection of your punches as you add slips and feints to your routine. Good boxers are never predictable. So mix it up!

Mirror Training

One of the best ways to perfect your punches and movement is to shadowbox in front of a mirror. You need a large mirror and sufficient space that allows you to punch and move freely. If a combination feels awkward and is not flowing you can check your performance in front of the mirror and make modifications. Are you holding your hands too low? Are your arms at the correct angle? Are you shifting your body weight properly and effortlessly? By studying your movement and punches in front of a mirror you will find it easier to make adjustments and change your execution and delivery. Throwing punches correctly allows for smooth transitions and reduces the chance of injuring your shoulder and elbow joints. Put time into practising shadowboxing and mirror training to ensure an easy transition to working on the bags.

Shadowboxing with Hand Weights

Once you have mastered your punches, practise your shadowboxing routine holding onto light hand weights, 1–1.5kg (2–3lb). This added resistance will remind you to keep your hands up to help develop muscle strength and endurance in your shoulders and arms. Only use hand weights once you are completely warmed up, and throw your punches no more than 60 per cent of your maximum punching power. Ensure you are executing the

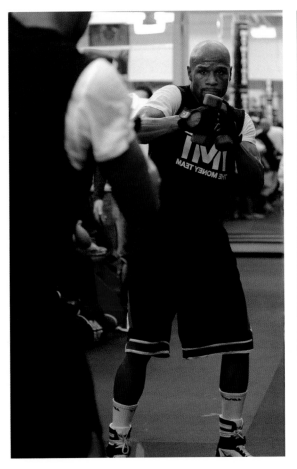

Mayweather Jr mirror training using hand weights.

Classic Shadowboxing Combinations

1. Double and triple jabs.
2. 'One–two': left jab followed by a straight right.
3. 'One–two–three': left jab, straight right, left hook.
4. 'One–two–three–four': left jab, straight right, left hook, right uppercut.
5. Left jab–right uppercut–left hook.
6. Left jab–left hook–straight right–left hook.
7. Jab–jab–right: a double left jab followed by a straight right.
8. Feint the left jab – throw a straight right – finish with a left hook.
9. Left jab to the body – left jab to the head.
10. 'One–two' to the body, 'one–two' to the head.

punches properly and have a secure grip on the weights. Do not use weights heavier than 1.5kg (3lb) as the excess load may pose an increased risk of injury to the ligaments and tendons of your joints.

To Start your Workout

After thoroughly warming up and completing one 3-minute round of shadowboxing without weights, perform one or two rounds while holding the hand weights. This will challenge you to keep your hands up high in the on-guard position and teach you to utilize proper punching technique. The arm and shoulder muscles will be challenged, resulting in improved muscular strength and endurance, giving you faster and more powerful punches.

Free Style Shadowboxing

Freestyle shadowboxing lets you practise all the punches and boxing moves. It allows you to develop your own individual style. Since you are not wearing boxing gloves or striking a bag, your hands will never feel faster or lighter than when you are shadowboxing. As you become proficient with the classic shadowboxing combinations, start to improvise offensive and defensive moves, develop smooth transitions, and add slips, ducks, and feints. Your goal is to deliver fast paced punches that flow easily and allow you to slip and counterpunch your opponent's moves.

Get in the zone by developing a boxer's mentality. Would you give any less than 100 per cent if you were facing a live opponent? Visualize doing battle in the ring, focus and give your best effort throughout your fitness boxing workout. Enjoy the freedom of movement and the opportunity to create countless punch combinations that will be limited only by your own imagination.

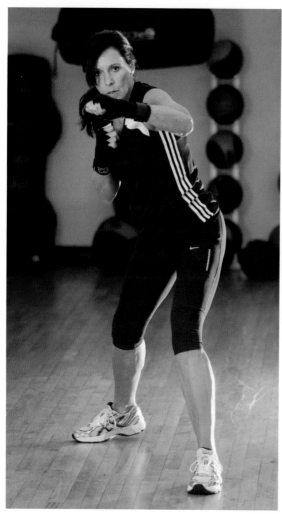

Getting in the zone.

your partner calls 'three', throw a left hook and when your partner calls 'four', throw a right uppercut. Always bring your hands quickly back to the on-guard position, move around and prepare for the next call.

Next, start to work on punch combinations. When a one-two is called, throw a left jab, followed by a straight right. For a one-two-three, throw a left jab, straight right, and then a left hook. For a one-two-three-four, throw a left jab, straight right, left hook, and end with a right uppercut.

When calling out punch sequences for your partner ensure there is adequate time for the puncher to move around between punch combinations. This exercise will teach you to react quickly and improve your response time.

Punch Sequencing Summary

'One': jab

'Two': straight right

'Three': left hook

'Four': right uppercut

'One-two': jab – straight right

'One-two-three': jab – straight right – left hook

'One-two-three-four': jab – straight right – left hook – right uppercut.

Always remember to return your hands to the on-guard position and keep moving around until your partner calls the next sequence. When it is your turn to call the punch sequence for your partner call out plenty of single jabs. Remember the jab should be the most frequently thrown punch. The purpose of this drill is to continuously punch and move, gradually building punch combinations.

SHADOWBOXING DRILLS

Basic Drill (3-minute round)

For this 3-minute drill you will need a training partner to call out some basic punch combinations and motivate you. As the round begins have your hands in the on-guard position, keep moving continuously and be ready to respond as your partner calls out single and multiple punch combinations. When your partner calls 'one', throw a left jab. When your partner calls 'two', throw a straight right. When

Speed-Punch Blitz (Intermediate to Advanced Drill)

Champion boxers will often throw 300 punches in a 3-minute round. Successful boxers condition themselves by constantly throwing punch after punch. This drill will give you a sense of what is like to throw multiple punches at maximum power. This is a conditioning drill that will definitely increase your heart rate quite quickly. It is important to be aware of proper punch execution.

Throw crisp punches for one minute to complete a circuit. This is accomplished by throwing a ten-punch flurry as fast as possible, taking a small break (2 seconds) in between the ten punches and repeat this a total of ten times. Remember to take deep breaths during the 2-second break, in between the flurry combinations.

Complete your first one-minute circuit throwing crisp punches. Take a 20-second rest before starting your second minute punch-flurry circuit. Aim to throw 100 punches in one minute. Take another 20-second rest and finish with a third round. Breathe naturally while throwing all of your punches and always ensure that you are not holding your breath. If you finish your 100 punches in under a minute just keep moving and jabbing until the minute is up. Focus on working multiple combinations throwing all your punches at full blast. During the 20-second rest perform shoulder circles to loosen up your shoulders and back.

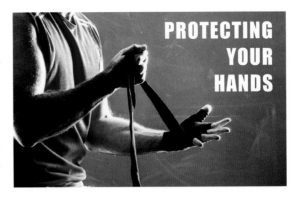

PROTECTING YOUR HANDS

Protecting your hands should be one of your highest priorities when performing a fitness boxing workout. Properly wrapping your hands and utilizing quality gloves is the way to start.

Hand Wraps

The purpose of hand wrapping is to protect the bones, joints, and ligaments in your hands, to give additional support to your wrists, and to avoid cuts to your knuckles. These reusable protective wraps reduce the chance of both short-term and long-term damage and discomfort to your hands.

There are basically two different styles of hand wraps. Mexican-style hand wraps are generally a blend of spandex and semi-elastic cotton that allows for a superior fit. Traditional hand wraps are made of a cotton woven material that tends to bunch and become heavy when your hands sweat.

Hand wraps are available in various lengths, 400–450cm (160–180in). If your hand wraps are too short you will be unable to wrap your hands effectively and thoroughly for protection. We recommend using the longer hand wraps at 450cm (180in). Also look for wraps with a wide Velcro closure for a more secure fit and durability.

There are many different techniques for wrapping your hands, each ritualistic to the individual. Some may want more wrap coverage around the knuckle area and others may want more wrap support on the wrist area. With practice you will make tweaks and little adjustments that will best suit your needs.

Speed-punch Drill

Perform this drill only after you are thoroughly warmed up.

Circuit 1 (1 minute) 10 sets of ten punches
Rest: 20 seconds
Circuit 2 (1 minute) 10 sets of ten punches
Rest: 20 seconds
Circuit 3 (1 minute) 10 sets of ten punches
Rest: 20 seconds

Depending on your conditioning level you can increase the difficulty level by holding onto hand weights. Since this is an intense punching drill use no more than 1kg (2lb) hand weights and remember to throw your punches at 60 per cent.

Never underestimate the importance of shadowboxing, not just as a warm-up or as a cool-down, but an important facet of your overall fitness boxing workout.

BASIC HAND WRAPPING TECHNIQUE

This is an effective hand wrapping method.

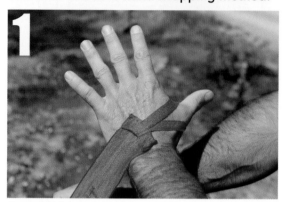

Step 1 With a relaxed open hand, spread your fingers wide. Place loop of the hand wrap around the thumb with the wrap falling to the front side of the hand.

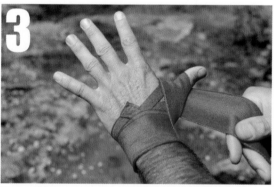

Step 2 Wrap twice around the wrist.

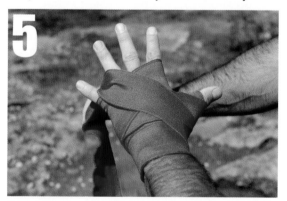

Step 3 Wrap once around the thumb. Always wrap in the direction away from the body.

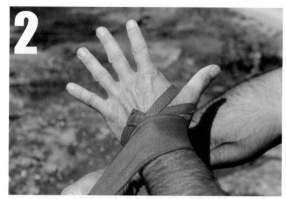

Step 4 Wrap around the knuckles three or four times and make sure you keep your fingers spread wide. Make a fist often to check that the tension of the hand wrap is not too tight. Overlap the side edges of the wrap slightly, keeping it flat.

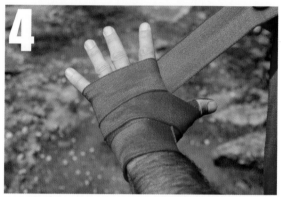

Step 5 Bring the wrap to the base of the thumb using it as the anchor. Pull the wrap between the small finger and the ring finger.

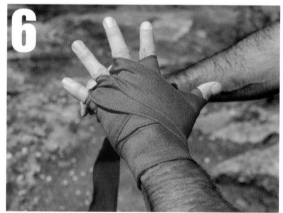

Step 6 Return the wrap to the base of the thumb and pull it between the ring finger and the long finger.

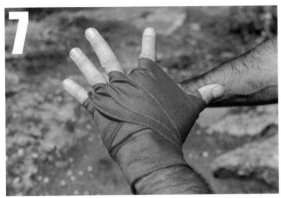

Step 7 Return to the base of the thumb once again and pull the wrap between the long finger and the index finger and then back to the wrist.

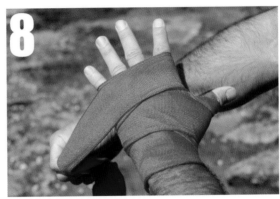

Step 8 From the wrist take the wrap to the knuckles and wrap a few more times.

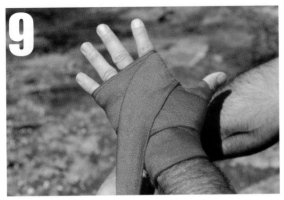

Step 9 With the remainder, continue to wrap around the wrist and hand in a figure of eight pattern. Pull the wrap in front and down toward the wrist.

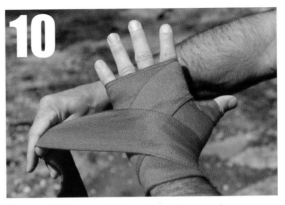

Step 10 Wrap under the wrist and up over the front of the hand to finish the second part of the figure of eight pattern. Repeat several times.

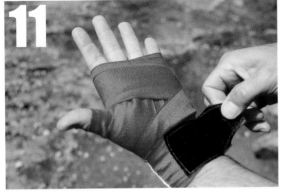

Step 11 Leave sufficient wrap to finish around the wrist a few times. Secure with the Velcro fastener.

It is important to wrap with an even tension. The wrap should feel snug enough to give sufficient support, but not so tight that your hand circulation is compromised. When you are training, always wear your hand wraps under your gloves to protect your hands, knuckles and wrists.

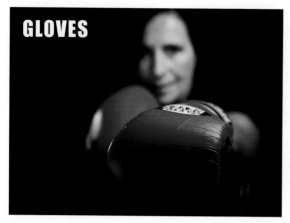

GLOVES

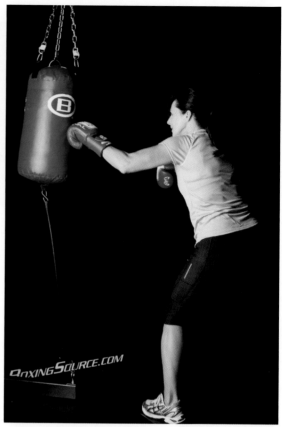

For boxing training there are three types of gloves: boxing gloves, sparring gloves and heavy bag gloves. Boxing gloves are used in competitive matches and are secured by laces. Sparring gloves are used for sparring and training drills and can either have Velcro fasteners or laces. Heavy bag gloves are used to hit the bags and focus mitts. They are secured with Velcro fasteners. Gloves should be used specifically for what they are designed for. Bag gloves should not be used for sparring or boxing.

Heavy bag gloves.

Heavy Bag Gloves

Heavy bag gloves are designed to hold up to the wear and tear of hitting a heavy bag and focus mitts versus hitting an opponent. For fitness boxing workouts you will need a quality pair of heavy bag gloves.

The gloves give extra protection for your hands, wrists, and knuckles. Ensure there is adequate space inside the gloves when your hands are wrapped, allowing for sufficient blood circulation. The gloves need to be snug around your hands and fit comfortably and feel secure. Velcro fasteners provide extra support for the wrists and make it easy to put the gloves on and off quickly. They are generally made of leather or synthetic materials. Many of the higher quality gloves also have sweat-wicking properties inside the glove.

Personal preference will dictate the weight of the glove you choose, ranging from 10 to 16 ounces. It is essential that your gloves feel comfortable and have sufficient padding to absorb the impact of hitting the heavy bag.

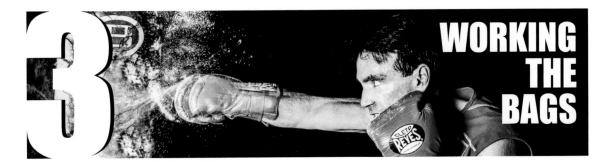

WORKING THE BAGS

The fitness industry is continually trying to create the latest and most sophisticated training equipment that promises remarkable results in the shortest time possible. Yet the simplicity in the design and effectiveness of the heavy bag, speed bag and double-end bag makes this 'old-school' training equipment timeless. You would be hard pressed to find a more dynamic training experience than working the bags.

Old School Meets New School

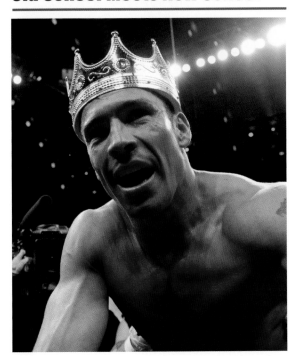

'Boxing had a primitive beginning, but has advanced into an intricate physical science of fighting. It has developed into more of a contest of skill, talent, and dedication.'
(Sergio Martinez, Champion)

The fitness boxing workout uses modern research and knowledge providing new drills, routines, and training techniques to create the most effective workout. The way the bags are used has been updated and revitalized. Working out on the heavy bag, speed bag and double-end bag provides immediate feedback with respect to your technique, ability and punching power. Striking the heavy bag provides an immense release of tension, and improves muscular strength and endurance. Hitting the speed bag develops quickness and hand-eye coordination. Punching the double-end bag tests and develops your agility and reaction time.

HEAVY BAG

The heavy bag has legendary status as one of the most important pieces of apparatus in preparing future world boxing champions. There is a great spontaneous creativity involved in hitting the heavy bag, with an endless number of punch combinations available. It is an exceptional workout that challenges your aerobic, anaerobic, and musculature systems. It is the most important piece of equipment for your fitness boxing workout.

The heavy bag is your opponent. There is really no other way to look at it. Treat it with respect, like a dangerous challenger that can strike you at any time. Remember, the sport we are trying to emulate is boxing, so visualization is extremely important. Move and throw punches on the bag as though you have a real live opponent in front of you. Warm up properly and prepare to go into battle with your virtual opponent, the heavy bag.

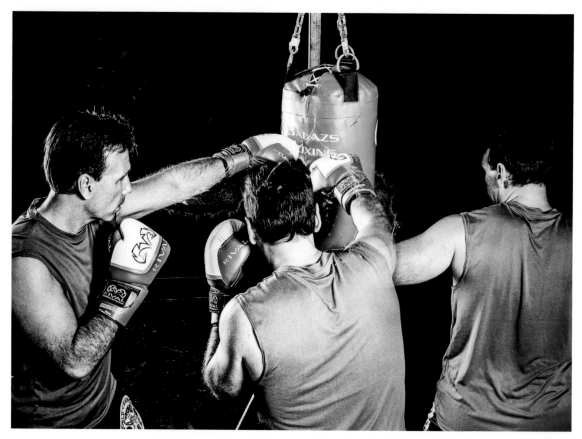

Throw punches with precision, passion and purpose.

The time you have put into your shadow boxing, mirror training, and practising the fundamentals will benefit your transition to the heavy bag. There is an old saying in boxing 'nothing stays still in the ring'. When working the heavy bag constantly move, slip and duck while throwing punch combinations. Work the bag as though you are competing in the boxing ring and throw punches with precision, passion, and purpose.

Technique vs Power

'Sometimes I just like to focus on the technique and get it done as perfectly as possible. Then sometimes you just want to hit the bag as hard as you can and beat it up.' (Cecilia Braekhus, Female World Welterweight Champion)

HEAVY BAG BASICS

Boxing Stance

After properly wrapping your hands and putting on your gloves, establish your boxing stance in front of the bag. Fully extend your left arm making contact with the knuckle portion of your glove on the bag. Keep the wrist straight. Take a step back, moving 15cm (6in) away from the bag. This is the starting distance for working the bag and throwing punches. The moment your fist makes contact with the heavy bag tighten your fist. Keep the hands in a semi-relaxed fist as you move around the bag, as constantly holding your fist tight and staying too tense will waste energy.

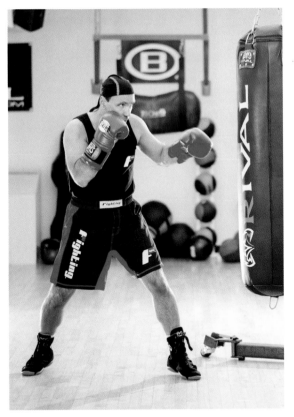

Hands on-guard, ready to punch.

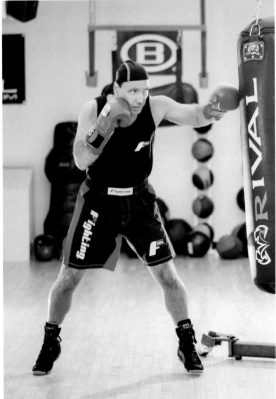

Your left jab is your range finder.

Create Space

Determine your maximum punching distance. Throw some jabs ensuring your arm is fully extended as your glove makes contact with the centre of the bag. Make sure you are not standing too close to the bag, keeping a realistic distance from your virtual or imaginary opponent. Your legs will move you into proper punch range. The aim is to maintain a consistent distance between you and the heavy bag.

Range

Be aware of your distance from the heavy bag, keeping it in view at all times. Move with the bag and stay slightly more than arm's length away. Your left jab is your range finder and it will give you a sense of how close you have to be to land other punches. Your straight punches will set up the short punches, such as hooks and uppercuts. Make use of your legs and footwork to move into range to strike the bag.

Proper Punching Technique

Focus on throwing crisp punches, aiming to hit the centre of the bag. When throwing jabs and straight rights, your arms should be almost fully extended upon impact. As soon as your glove makes impact with the bag, quickly return your fists to the on-guard position ready to throw your next punch. Your punch should jolt the bag with a quick snapping motion. If you leave the punch out there too long, you are pushing the bag resulting in a sloppy, lazy punch. Keep your neck, shoulders, and arms relaxed and this will assist in throwing fast snapping punches. 'Lead with speed, follow with power.' Do not sacrifice technique for punching power. Start by throwing light, quick punches, gradually adding more power. Use your imagination as you build two- and three-punch combinations.

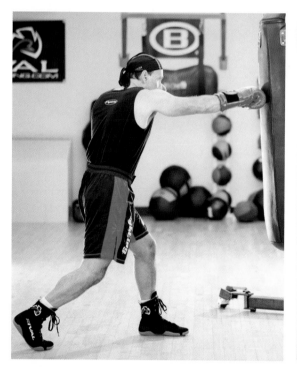

Straight right.

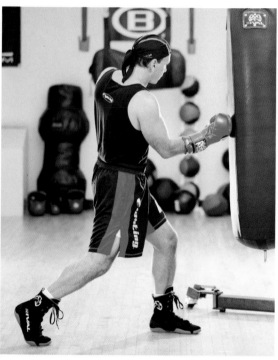

Right uppercut on the heavy bag.

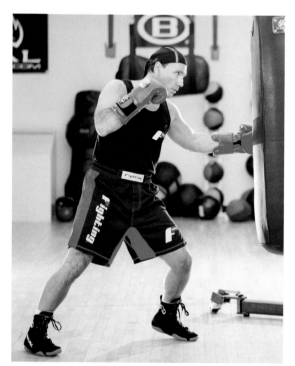

Left hook to the mid-section of the bag.

Movement

As you continue to establish your range and move around the bag, step forward with your punches and then step backward. This is called 'punch and get out'. At the moment of impact, keep your core muscles tight and return your hands to the on-guard position quickly. Pivot on the balls of your feet when throwing punches to maintain balance. This provides a stable stance from which maximum power can be executed. Never stand flat-footed; always stay on the balls of your feet ready to move in any direction. Once you have found your range with your left jab, try throwing some straight rights, and one-two combinations. Incorporate the slight swinging motion of the bag into your punching rhythm.

Natural Swinging Motion

The heavy bag will swing in a natural motion when it is hit properly. You want to use this motion to time your punches while you move around the bag. Coordinate your footwork with the swinging motion of the bag and time

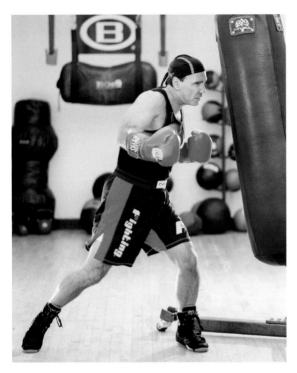

Move with the natural swinging motion of the bag.

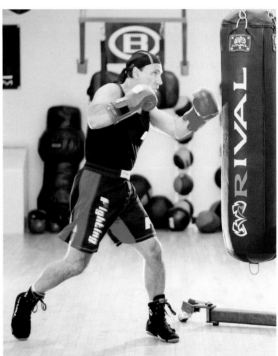

Find a consistent punching pace.

your strikes by ensuring that your punches make contact with the bag as it comes toward you. Pushing your punches and not snapping them will create unnecessary swinging of the bag. Throwing wild punches or whaling at the bag as it is moving away will also cause the bag to swing uncontrollably, and you will never develop a good rhythm. A technically correct crisp punch will jolt the bag but not make it move excessively.

Stay Focused

Your focus is to maintain proper punching form and work hard throughout the entire round. Sustain a good punching pace for the entire 3 minutes of every round and use your 1-minute rest to recover between rounds. When performing this type of interval training, you may have a tendency to hit the bag vigorously for the first 30–40 seconds and then be too winded to continue punching for the remainder of round. Real boxing matches do not have long periods of inactivity so stay busy

and keep moving to emulate a real fight situation. Find a consistent punching pace that you can continue with and persevere to the end of the round.

Breathe Correctly

The body tenses up while punching the heavy bag and there is often a tendency to hold your breath for a split second. Stay relaxed and exhale as you throw your punches, then breathe in to get a new supply of oxygen to your working muscles. Exhaling correctly is necessary in order to perform aerobic activities and will allow for more power to each punch.

When watching a boxer training or in an actual fight, you will notice that the boxer makes a quick sniffing sound as they punch. This exhalation of the breath is referred to as the 'snort'. Boxers are taught to keep their mouths closed and exhale through their nose when throwing punches in case they are hit in the jaw. Boxers also feel that by breathing this way they can deliver their punches with more power, however there is no scientific; research that this works. The point is for you to find a natural breathing rhythm that suits you. Exhale on exertion and then inhale to replenish the oxygen to the body.

Mix It Up

Vary the tempo, speed and selection of your punch combinations. Visualize punches coming at you from an opponent, slip or duck, and then counter with your own punches. Slipping and ducking helps you develop torso strength and improve your balance. Make sure you are not just targeting the head area. Throw some body punches into the mix. Set up your hooks and uppercuts with your straight punches. Move into position, throw your power shots and move out. Stay busy, find a smooth rhythm, and throw 'punches in bunches'.

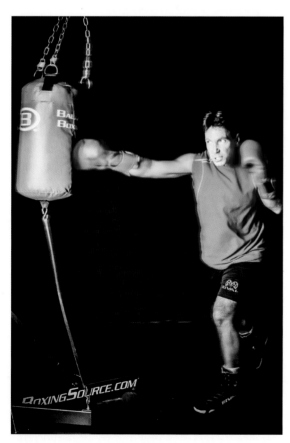

Throw punches in bunches.

Key Points: Heavy Bag

- Focus on proper execution and punching technique.
- Establish a realistic distance from the bag, slightly more than a jab's distance away. Your arm should be almost fully extended on impact when throwing straight punches.
- Nothing stays still in the ring. Make sure you move around while throwing punches.
- Snap your punches to avoid excessive swing of the heavy bag. Time your punches to make contact with the bag as it moves slightly toward you.
- Do not drop your hands after punching. This will leave you out of position for your next series of punches.

DEFENSIVE MOVES

Why should you incorporate defensive moves into heavy bag training? Blending your punch combinations with defensive moves adds another dimension of realism to your fitness boxing workout. By adding slipping and ducking moves your core and leg muscles will be physically challenged.

Visualization

As mentioned, visualizing an opponent keeps the workout interesting and will motivate you to work harder. Some of these defensive moves will also be featured in the focus mitt drills (Chapter 4).

Slipping

If you have been practising your slips while shadowboxing it should be easy to incorporate them into your heavy bag routine. With

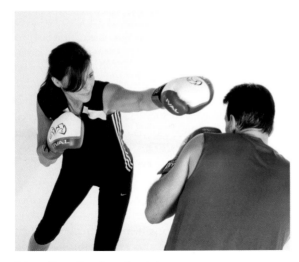

Visualize slipping the jab.

your hands in the protective position imagine your opponent throwing a left jab. Slip the punch by dipping to your right, making sure your eyes are always on your opponent. After slipping you can counter with a right to the body. Slip a straight right by bending your knees and lowering your body to the left. Counter by throwing a left hook.

Ducking

Ducking is another defensive move with great fitness benefits engaging the gluteals, quadriceps and core muscles. Use your legs to lower

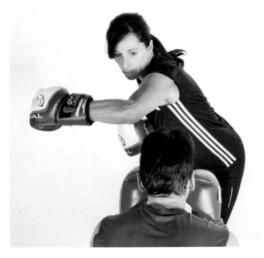

Visualize ducking under a left hook.

your body and move under a punch. The body shifts from one side to the other. When you duck under a punch and to the left, counter back with a left hook and when you duck under and over to the right, counter with a right hook.

Blocking

There is no real fitness benefit to blocking, but it does help create actual combat scenarios. Keeping your hands up high in the on-guard position and your gloves against your head, imagine your opponent throwing a left hook. Block the punch with your right glove. You can throw a left hook counter punch to the bag. Blocking a straight right from your opponent with your left glove will allow you to counter with a right uppercut to the body.

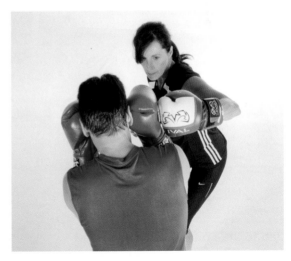

Visualize blocking a punch.

HEAVY BAG PUNCH COMBINATIONS

Basic Combinations
Double and Triple Jabs

Throw two or three rapid-fire jabs. Do not worry about power when throwing double and triple jabs. Execute a stronger first jab to set up the location and follow with the second or third jab by flicking fast and light. There is no pause between the jabs. The second and third jabs are executed by pulling back approximately one-third the distance of the first jab. It is all about speed, moving your opponent off-balance, and setting up to throw more powerful punches.

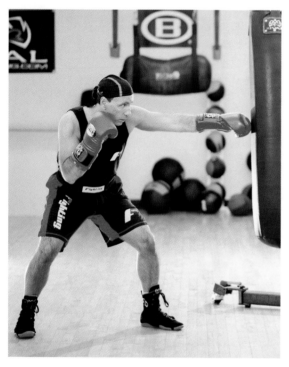

Bend your knees to throw body punches.

Jab to the Body – Jab to the Head

Lower your body position and step forward as you launch a quick left jab to the body. Now raise your body position and immediately launch a jab to the head region. After you land your second jab, quickly step away from the bag ready to throw your next combination. When throwing body punches aim dead centre just below the mid-portion of the bag.

The One-Two

This classic punch sequence is utilized more than any other combination. Throw a fast left jab followed immediately by a powerful straight right. Ensure both hands quickly return to the on-guard position. Move away from the bag ready to throw your next combination.

Throw one-twos to the head and one-twos to the body. To throw a one-two combination to the body, bend your legs to lower your position and aim your punches to the mid-section of the bag. Throwing body punches from an upright position means you are throwing on a downward angle, reducing the effectiveness of the punch, and leaving you open. Ensure your hands are in the correct on-guard position.

One – Two – Hook

Move forward as you launch a quick one-two combination (left jab, straight right). You should now be in position to throw a short left hook to complete the combination. Move away from the bag and get ready to throw your next punch sequence.

Double Jab to the Body (Single Jab to the Head – Straight Right – Left Hook)

Lower your body throwing two quick, light jabs to the mid-section of the bag. Move up and throw a hard jab to the head, followed by a straight right to the head. Pivot and throw a short left hook to the head.

Jab to the Head – Slip Right – Straight Right – Left Hook to the Body

Lead with a left jab to the head. Visualize a left jab coming from your opponent and slip to the right. Immediately come back with a straight right to the head and dig in with a left hook to the body. Make sure your hands are up when you slip, remembering to pivot on the balls of your feet shifting your weight to add power to your punches.

Jab – Right Uppercut – Left Hook – Short Right Hand

Fire a left jab to the head, move forward and throw a right uppercut to the body, followed by a left hook to the head and then finish with a short right to the head.

Intermediate/Advanced Combinations

One – Two – Double Left Hook

Lower your body position and throw a quick one-two to the mid-section. Follow up with a fast left hook to the body and immediately rise up and throw your second left hook to the head. Both hooks need to be in quick succession without a pause.

Feint Jab – Straight Right – Left Hook – Straight Right

With your left fist, appear to throw the left jab, hold back, and then launch your right hand to the head instead. Next throw a left hook to the head and finish with a straight right to the head. As mentioned earlier feints are designed to fool your opponent. Feints make it appear that you are going to throw one punch, but you throw a different punch. They have to be quick, subtle and realistic. Incorporate feints into your other punch combinations.

Punch Flurries

Flurries are light, crisp, fast punches thrown in bunches. Generally throw four to six rapid-fire punches at a time. The delivery is fast so there is little time to load up on your punches. Just let your hands go.

Theme Your Heavy Bag Rounds

In Round 1, visualize an elusive opponent who is constantly moving while throwing punches at you. When faced with this type of opponent plan your punches strategically. Throw plenty of jabs to set up your power punches. In the next round visualize an opponent who likes to attack and place pressure on you. Slip, pivot, duck and throw counter punches in this defensive round. Next round, imagine you are an inside fighter throwing hooks and inside combinations. Step closer to the bag and use power behind your punches.

If you have a favourite boxer, imagine you are stepping into the ring with them. Visualize their unique fighting style and counter their offensive attack with effective movement and punch combinations.

Key Points: Combinations

- Work the bag like you are in the ring.
- Develop your punch combinations so they follow a logical order and leave you on balance.
- Move around and incorporate the natural swinging motion of the bag into your workout.
- Add slips and ducks while working the bag.
- To facilitate smooth movement stay on the balls of your feet. Never stand flat-footed.

HEAVY BAG DRILLS

The drills described here are a great way to finish off your heavy bag workout. Ensure you are properly warmed-up before you perform any of these drills and try to include at least one of these drills into your fitness boxing workout. As you become better conditioned, add two or three of the drills at the end of your workout.

Heavy Bag Ladder Drill

This drill involves throwing rapid-fire straight punches and moving around the bag briefly before starting your next punch sequence.

Ladder 1

Start by throwing 12 sharp jabs as fast as possible. Move around the bag for about five to 8 seconds keeping your hands up and changing direction often. Then move into range and throw 11 crisp jabs. Move around again briefly and throw 10 jabs. Reduce the number of jabs you throw by one each time, continuing down the ladder until you throw just one jab. This is the end of your first ladder. Take a 1-minute rest.

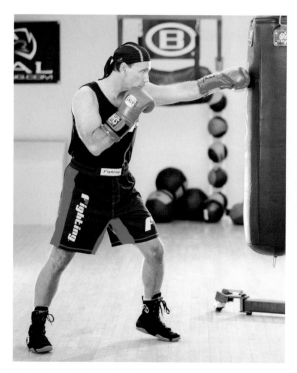

Ladders – Throw rapid-fire jabs.

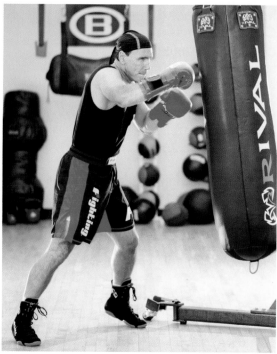

Speed sprints – punch as fast as you can.

Ladder 2

Start your second ladder by throwing one-two punch combinations (left jab–straight right). Throw 12 one-twos, move changing direction, and then launch 11 one-twos and so on until you throw just 1 one-two punch combination.

Punching Speed Sprints

Some of our drills are more condition-based rather than skill or technical based. Sprint training is definitely a conditioning drill that challenges your upper body musculature and your cardio-respiratory system for maximum fitness output. Punching speed sprints are a succession of fast punches delivered for a specific amount of time and followed by a brief rest. Punch as many times as you can for a short burst, rest, and then repeat the process again. This sprint recreates the maximum punch-speed and recovery ratio that are so important in a fight situation.

Since there is no footwork involved, you do not have to be in your boxing stance for this drill. Face the bag straight on with both arms at an equal reach distance. Get into a position that allows your arms to be fully extended at impact. Maintain this distance throughout the entire drill and hold your core tight. Shift the body weight slightly forward on the balls of your feet with your knees relaxed. Hit the bag with a one-two, one-two rhythm without any pauses. This is non-stop, rapid fire punching. Keep your breathing steady throughout the sprints.

Sprint for 15 seconds, take a 15-second rest and repeat two more times. As your conditioning improves, increase your sprinting time by 5-second increments working up to 30-second sprints. Keep your rest intervals the same length as your sprint intervals. Since your heart rate is elevated keep moving and walking around during the rest interval. It is important to remember to maintain a regular breathing rhythm when performing the sprints. Use your watch timer or a partner to indicate the sprint times. Perform the sprint sequence three to four times.

Sample Beginner Speed Sprint

Sprint 1: 15 seconds Rest: 15 seconds

Sprint 2: 15 seconds Rest: 15 seconds

Sprint 3: 15 seconds Rest: 15 seconds

Dirty 30s

This challenging three-part drill is broken down into 30-second intervals and repeated twice in a 3-minute round.

1st 30 seconds: Box and Move

In your boxing stance, punch the heavy bag at a fast pace, moving and throwing quick combinations as you circle the bag. Mix up your punches by throwing a variety of jabs, hooks, crosses, and body shots.

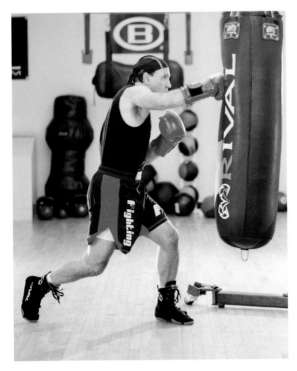

Dirty 30s – box and move.

2nd 30 seconds: High Knee Run and Punching

Face the bag straight on. Punch the heavy bag non-stop with both hands while running on the spot, lifting your knees high.

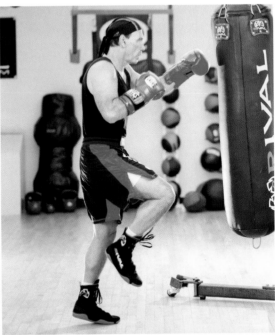

Throw punches with both hands.

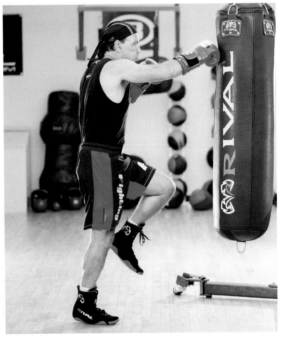

Lift your knees high.

3rd 30 seconds: Knockout!

Return to your boxing stance and hit the bag full force as if you are trying to knock out your opponent. Throw as many punches as possible, using proper technique, leverage and rotation.

Repeat this drill twice to complete the 3-minute round.

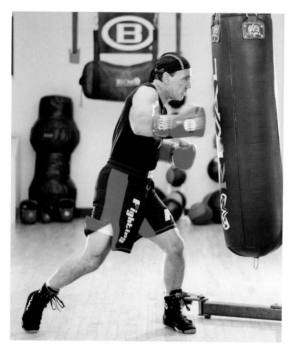

Dirty 30s – knockout punches.

Punch and Push-Up Drill

Alternate throwing a crisp one-two combination on the heavy bag, then immediately drop down and perform one push-up. Quickly jump up into your boxing stance and perform another one-two combination. This sequence will really fatigue your upper body and shoulder muscles. Maintain correct punching form followed by properly executed push-ups. Push-ups are performed with your gloves on. Focus on keeping your wrists straight and strong, your body weight centred through the knuckle portion of the gloves, and your body held straight and tight. Ensure you are not holding your breath, especially when performing your push-ups as

your heart rate will be elevated. Exhale on exertion. Repeat the punch and push-up sequence for 1 minute.

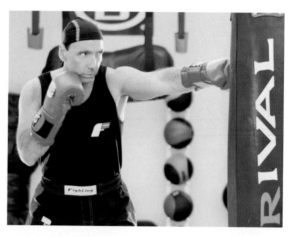

Punch and Push-up Drill – jab.

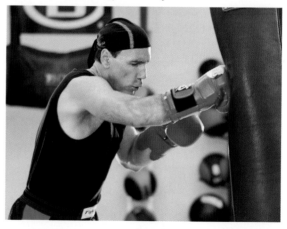

Straight right.

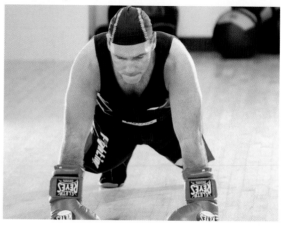

Push-up – up position.

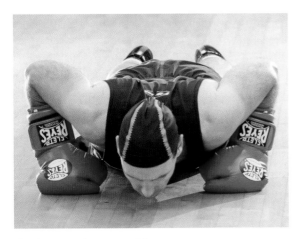

Push-up – down position.

If you have difficulty performing a full-body push-up, you can modify the push-up by placing both of your knees on the floor.

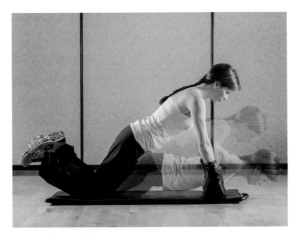

Modified push-up.

Types of Heavy Bag

Whether you are training at home, at a fitness club or working out at a boxing club there are numerous styles and sizes of heavy bags specific to your training requirements.

Material and Filling

Synthetic, vinyl-coated bags can take a pounding, but we find high quality leather bags are the most durable. The firmness of the bag will depend on both the internal packing density and the exterior material. For home use it is worthwhile to spend a bit more and purchase a high-quality heavy bag.

Hanging Bag

Depending on your needs and experience, your weight, height and punching strength will influence the size of the bag you purchase. A good starting size for the average person is a 30kg (70lb) hanging bag. Hanging bags weigh from 20kg (50lb) to 110kg (250lb). The heavier ones move less and are also less forgiving and more jarring when hit.

Floor Bag

Floor bags can weigh up to 180kg (400lb). This added weight is needed to keep the bag from tipping when being punched. They are fairly portable and easily placed in an exercise area and can be purchased at most sports stores. The disadvantage of a floor bag is the absence of the swinging motion that you get from a hanging bag, which forces you to move with the bag and time your strikes.

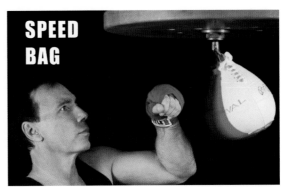

The rhythmic sounds of the speed bag reverberate through the air when you walk into any boxing club. That familiar rat-a-tat-tat cadence is unique to this brilliant, old piece of training equipment and creates a distinctive and inspiring sound.

Punching with speed and accuracy is easy when you can stop anytime you feel like it. In the ring though, you are always being forced to punch even when you are exhausted. The speed bag challenges your upper body endurance and forces you to continue punching when your arms are becoming fatigued. You must also focus and concentrate on keeping the bag moving properly. Eye-hand coordination is developed, and with practice striking the speed bag just at the correct time becomes second nature.

At first, attempting to hit the speed bag can be exceptionally frustrating but ultimately the rewards are worthwhile. Stick with it and the results will be faster punches, upper body and shoulder development, and improved hand-eye coordination.

Adjusting the Speed Bag

Speed bags are suspended below a horizontal platform connected by a swivel, allowing for a free rotational movement. The exterior is made of stitched leather and it is filled with an air bladder. Available in various sizes, the smaller bags are approximately 10cm (8in) long; they move fast and rebound quickly, making them a greater challenge to hit. The largest speed bags are around 20cm (14in) long; they react slower and are easier to hit than the smaller bags.

The bottom of the speed bag should be eye level if you are using a small speed bag. For a larger speed bag, the bag should be one to two inches above your chin. Some speed bag platforms are adjustable so the bag can be moved to the appropriate level for you.

Check to see how much air is in the bag. It needs to be firm, but not rock hard. If you are having difficulty hitting the bag, letting some of the air out of the bladder will slow down the bag movement and allow you to hit it more easily.

Hitting the Speed Bag

Triplet Rhythm

The rhythm of hitting the speed bag is called a triplet rhythm as the bag rebounds three times, forward-backward-forward, with each strike. So the sequence is 'strike one-two-three'. With the first strike, the bag moves away and hits the back portion of the platform (1).

It then rebounds and hits the front portion of the platform (2). The bag rebounds away once again to hit the back portion of the platform (3). This is the precise moment you strike the bag once again.

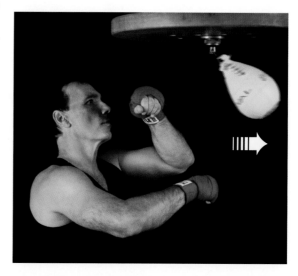

Bag hits back of platform.

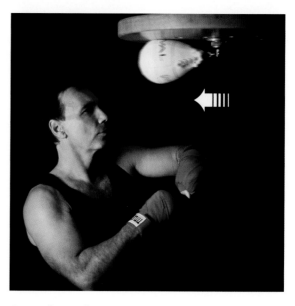

Bag rebounds.

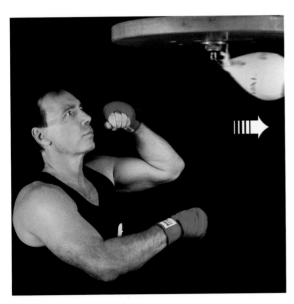

Ready to strike the bag again.

Proper Form

Step 1. Stand facing square to the bag with both shoulders equal distance from the bag. You do not have to be in the boxer's stance. Bring both fists up in front of your face, your arms bent and the elbows bent at about ninety degrees and tucked in by the sides of your body. Your fists are approximately 15–20cm (6–8in) away from the bag.

Step 2. Strike the bag in the centre, making sure your knuckles land flush against the leather. Hit straight through the bag. Ensure you are not 'chopping' at the bag with your strikes. Instead visualize hitting through the bag. Once you strike the bag, immediately circle your fist back to the starting position.

Step 3. Repeat striking the bag with the 'strike 1-2-3' rhythm remembering to keep both hands up by your face. It is often the transition from striking with one hand to using the other that breaks your rhythm and causes ineffective hits. Start with six to eight strikes with one hand until you get competent. Switch to the other hand. Everyone has a dominant hand, so stick with it until both hands are functioning equally. Reduce the number of repetitions to four hits, down to two, and then singles.

Step 4. Single strikes. As you make contact with the bag with one hand the opposite hand immediately comes up ready to strike the bag. Repeat, keeping this semi-circular movement concise and fast. As your punch speed increases, the circular range of motion that your arm goes through will become shorter. The single strike is more challenging, as the faster pace requires you to react sooner.

Focus Your Strikes

The area where your knuckles make contact on the bag and how hard you strike it will affect your ability to keep the bag under control. The bag will jam if you make contact too soon causing a clumsy rhythm. If you strike the bag too late, your fist will hit the underside of the bag. When starting out use medium force until you have mastered the punching rhythm.

Listen to the Rhythm

As you make faster contact with the bag it will be more difficult to see the rebounds, but you will still be able to hear the sounds. The triplet sequence has a distinct sound and paying attention to these sounds will assist you in developing a smooth punching rhythm. The first sound is the bag hitting the back of the platform after you strike it. The second sound is the bag moving forward and hitting the front of the platform. The third sound is the rebound of the bag moving away from you and hitting the back of the platform once again.

As you become more proficient increase your punch speed. Wearing hand wraps provides sufficient protection for your knuckles when striking the speed bag; however if your want more protection for your hands use speed bag striking mitts. These mitts have a flat punching surface and are lightly padded for extra protection.

Open Hand Method

If you are having difficulty controlling the speed bag, you can use the open-hand method to improve your technique. Address the bag straight-on so both hands have equal reach. Keep your hands open, your palms facing the bag and drive the centre of the bag forward with your open hand. Spreading the fingers wide allows for more contact time with the bag and better control. Allow the bag to roll off of your fingers in a straight swinging motion. Follow through bringing your hands straight back. This open handed method will help slow down the pace for beginners and get use to the 'strike 1-2-3' rhythm. Follow Steps 1-4 with open hands.

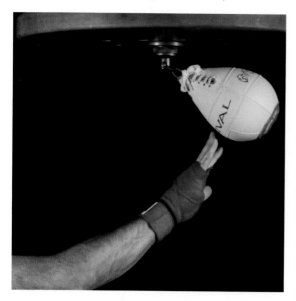

Open Hand Method – allow the bag to roll off your fingers.

Speed Bag Combinations

Four Strikes
Four strikes with each hand allows you to get a rhythm established before you switch to the other hand. A great way to start!

Double Strikes
Reducing down to double strikes means you are bringing your other hand into play sooner.

Single Strikes
Strike alternating hands. The transition from your right fist to your left fist is quick and needs to be smooth.

Strikes with Movement
Alternate strikes with each hand, while circling the platform. Try to keep the bag steady as you are moving.

Free-Style
Effortlessly go from multiple strikes to single strikes varying your speed and rhythm. This can include short bursts of rapid fire punching for 15–20 seconds and then back to a regular pace. Mix it up.

Key Points: Speed Bag

- Assume the standard speed bag stance, with your feet about shoulder width apart. Have your body facing the bag straight on to ensure that both arms have equal reach.
- Strike the bag moving your arms in small circles.
- Bring your fists back up to striking level after hitting the bag. Keeping your hands low will throw your timing off.
- Hit the bag lightly to maintain control.
- Make contact with the belly of the speed bag, not too high nor too low.

Use a smaller speed bag to challenge and improve your agility and eye-hand coordination. Vary the speed of the punches, with slower punches interspersed with sprints. Once you have your rhythm down, move around the bag while punching.

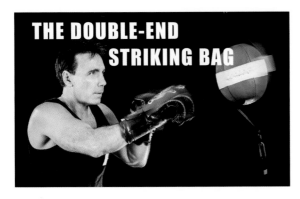

THE DOUBLE-END STRIKING BAG

The rebounding action of the double-end striking bag simulates the movement of an actual opponent. This improves reaction time and forces you to quickly make small adjustments to your punch execution and defensive moves. When you strike the double-end bag, it rebounds backward and forward in a random manner.

Sometimes referred to as a floor-to-ceiling ball, double-end bags are round, lightweight, inflatable sacks made of leather that are suspended vertically by a bungee or shock cord from the ceiling and anchored to the floor. They come in various sizes with the smaller bags being the most challenging to hit. How quickly the bag rebounds and how far it swings are also influenced by the tension of the shock cords.

Working on the double-end bag improves the speed and accuracy of your punch combinations. It also allows you to work on defensive techniques, such as slipping, without a partner. Save your power for the heavy bag, as the intention behind this multi-purpose piece of equipment is to challenge your coordination, reactions, timing and agility.

It is best to wear bag gloves when hitting the double-end bag. Gloves give you more control because of the larger contact surface and they also protect your hands. When you strike the double-end bag it will move quickly away, then rebound back at you. Keep your hands in the on-guard position and your gloves held firmly in front of your head. This will prevent the bag from making contact with your face. Either counter with a punch or slip out of the way.

Starting Out

Start in the orthodox boxing stance, hands up, and more than a jab's length away from the bag. Ensure you are far enough away from the bag so the bag will not rebound and hit you. It is from this position that you want to execute some jabs. Study how the bag rebounds back at you, at what angle and the speed it travels. It may seem as though the bag has a mind of its own.

Aim for the centre of the bag. If the bag is spiralling off to one side, you are not catching it dead centre. The movement of the bag should be forward and backward without any side-to-side motion when you strike it. Initially develop a sense of timing and discover how the bag reacts to your single straight punches (a left jab and a straight right) before moving onto combinations.

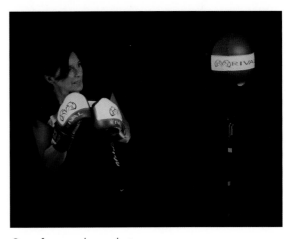

Stay focused, ready to move.

Basic Punch Combinations

Double Jabs

Throw two quick jabs. The second jab catches the bag on the rebound. Reset and then repeat the double jab.

One-two Combo

Throw a quick one-two (left jab–straight right). As your jab makes impact quickly throw your straight right before the bag fully rebounds. Throwing a one-two is trickier because you must react faster. Work on developing a smooth transition from the left to the right hand, always aiming for the centre of the bag.

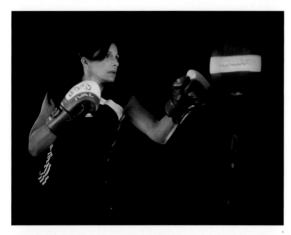

Aim for the centre of the bag.

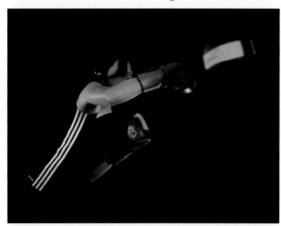

Execute crisp punches.

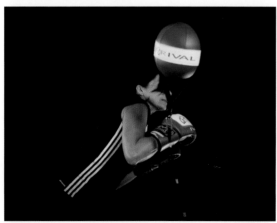

Maintain eye contact with the bag when slipping.

One-two – One-two

Move up to a four-punch combination. Left–right – left–right. Hit the bag in the same spot with each punch, ensuring you are not pausing between the punches. Try to strike with consistency to keep the bag under control. Stay on balance. Quickly land your four punches, reset and repeat. Repeat this rapid-fire sequence for 60 seconds.

Left-Left-Right/Right-Right-Left

This six-punch combination requires you to focus on light, fast punches emphasizing technique, not power. Throw two quick strikes with your left hand and follow with a short right. Immediately throw two quick rights followed by a left jab. Finish the six-punch combination, take a slight pause and repeat. If you are having difficulty with this combination, break it into two parts. Practise the first part of the sequence, left–left–right, over and over until you have the bag under control. Then work on the second half, right–right–left. Finally put the full six-punch sequence together. Repeat for 1-2 minutes.

Try these basic slip combinations:

Jab and Slip

Snap a left jab. As the bag starts to rebound quickly slip to the right, and then move back into position ready to throw your next punch. This drill simulates an incoming jab. When slipping, keep your hands up, elbows in and eyes on the bag. Ensure your core muscles are held tight and you shift your body weight over to the right side. Repeat practising the jab and slip until you develop your rhythm.

One-two – Slip

Launch a quick one-two combination. Just as your straight right makes contact with the bag, slip to the left. The rebound of the bag simulates an opponent's straight right coming at you. Keep your eyes on the bag and move out of the way. Return to the on-guard position to throw another one-two.

Key Points: Double End Bag

- Keep your fists up by your chin, elbows close to your body and eyes on the target.
- Focus on striking the bag flush and dead centre.
- Throwing hard, wild punches on the double-end bag will cause it to move erratically. Instead strike the bag with light, crisp, punches. This will enable you to develop a smooth punch rhythm.
- Save the power and strength for the heavy bag.
- When slipping, practise moving your head and shoulders just enough to avoid the rebound of the bag. If the slips are over-exaggerated, it will throw you off-balance and put you out of position to counterpunch effectively.
- Maintain a balanced stance staying on the balls of your feet.

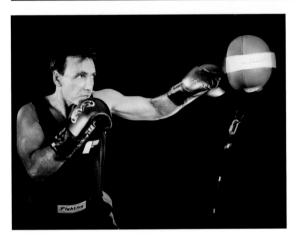

Develop creative combinations.

Freestyle on the Double-End Bag

In order to develop your timing and rhythm, dedicate several rounds working on the double-end bag. Remember this is the one piece of equipment that imitates sparring against a live opponent. The constant movement of the bag simulates an opponent moving and changing direction, and the rebound action replicates oncoming punches. Master your footwork, directional changes and rapid-fire punches, developing creative combinations and defensive moves. Training on the double-end bag results in quick reflexes and fast movements, and when combined with heavy bag and speed-bag training completes your training regimen.

ADDITIONAL EQUIPMENT

Other pieces of boxing equipment that you may want to incorporate into your training are the hanging uppercut bag and the uppercut-and-hook, wall-mounted bag.

Uppercut Bag

The uppercut is one of the most difficult punches to land effectively, and the uppercut bag is a great piece of equipment that allows you to develop this inside or close-range punch. The uppercut bag is basically a heavy bag hung horizontally. The angle of the bag allows you to execute uppercuts effectively.

Face the bag in your on-guard stance, knees bent and abdominal muscles held tight. As your fist makes contact with the bag ensure the knuckle portion of your glove is flush against the underside of the bag. Practise throwing left and right uppercuts. To land a left uppercut, shift your weight slightly to the left side, elbow tucked in by the side of your body and your knees bent. To land a right uppercut, shift your weight slightly to the right side, elbow in and knees bent. Try throwing a left and a right uppercut together, bending your knees and shifting your weight from side to side. Put three uppercuts together, remembering to transfer your weight from one side to the other side. Throw a left–right–left uppercut sequence, pause, and then a right–left–right uppercut

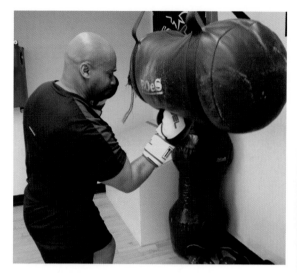

Practise throwing left and right uppercuts.

sequence, increasing your punch speed and power. Do not to wind up or pull back your arms before throwing your uppercuts.

You can effectively work on combinations that include uppercuts, hooks and straight punches. Use the underside of the bag for uppercuts, the end of the bag for hooks and the centre of the bag for your straight punches. Straight punches set up your short punches, so you want to practise standing far enough away from the uppercut bag to throw effective straight punches and then move in closer to land your uppercuts. Move back out before you start another combination. Add hooks to your sequences by using either end of the bag. Stand off to the right side of the bag to throw a right hook. Stand off to the left side of the bag to throw a left hook.

Try These Basic Uppercut Combinations:
Combination 1: Jab – Jab – Uppercut
In your boxing stance in front of the bag, throw two quick left jabs as you move forward. Immediately follow with a short right uppercut. Repeat.

Combination 2: One – Two – Uppercut
Start by throwing a one-two combination (left-jab and straight right). After your right hand has landed you should be in the correct posi-

tion to throw a short left uppercut. Quickly move away and repeat. Build onto this combination by adding a right uppercut (one – two – left uppercut – right uppercut).

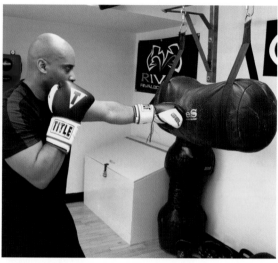

Straight punches set up your short punches.

Combination 3: Hook – Uppercut
Stand off to the right side of the bag and throw a right hook, followed by a left uppercut. Turn your body and pivot off your front foot as you throw the right hook and then drive off your rear foot as you launch the left uppercut. Change ends and throw a left hook followed by a right uppercut.

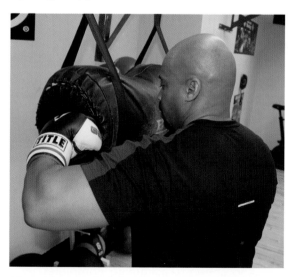

Use either end of the bag to practise hooks.

Key Points: Uppercut Bag

- Make sure your gloves land flush against the bag. Keep your elbows in by the sides of your body as you drive the punch straight up, striking with your knuckles.
- Bend your knees and lower your body driving the punch upward and into the bag.
- Keep the uppercut punch fast and tight. Do not make a large arm movement by winding up to throw the punch.

The Hook-and-Uppercut Wall Bag

The unique design of wall-mounted bags gives you the opportunity to practise punches from a variety of angles, especially hooks and uppercuts. Practise throwing punch combinations while you move in and out of position. Aim for the circular body and head target zones on the front and sides of the bag. This is a great piece of equipment to develop and perfect your short-range punches.

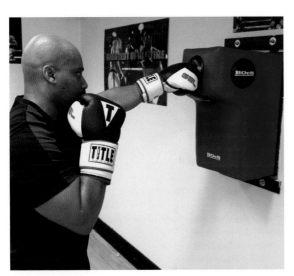

Aim for the circular target zones.

Here are Basic Hook-and-Uppercut Combinations:

Combination 1: Jab to the Body – Jab to the Head – Left Hook – Short Right

Launch a quick jab to the mid-section of the bag, followed by a jab to the head area. Finish with a hook to the left side of the bag and a short right to the front of the bag.

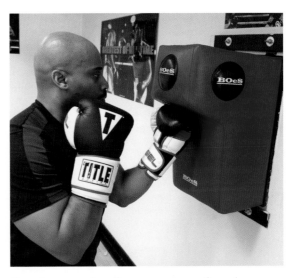

Practise punches from a variety of angles.

Combination 2: Jab Feint – Straight Right – Left Hook – Right Uppercut

Feint with your left jab, move forward as you throw the right lead, followed by a short left hook, then finish with a right uppercut.

Combination 3: One – Two – Left Hook – Right Uppercut

Throw a one-two (left jab–straight right) to the body. Follow with a left hook to the head zone and finish with a right uppercut. Remember to bend your knees to lower your body when throwing body punches.

Key Points: Hook/Uppercut Bag

- Punch and get out. The wall bag is the only bag that is stationary so you will not get the swinging motion. Constantly move in and out of position while throwing your punches.
- Ensure your punches land cleanly in the target zones and not on the outer edges of the bag.

The unique qualities of the various punching bags challenge your fitness capabilities and mental focus, develops your skill levels and your physicality. Always execute your punches and movement utilizing proper technique. If you make this commitment to challenge yourself, improvements in timing, eye-hand coordination, agility, speed and power can be achieved.

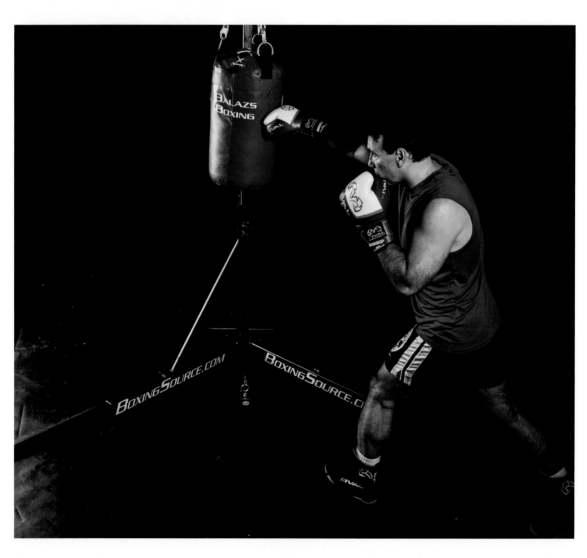

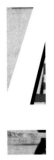
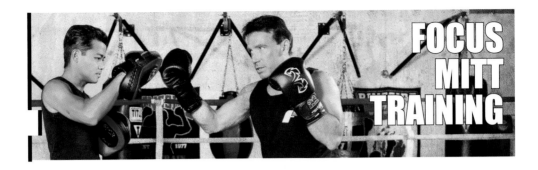

When you watch great boxers train with focus mitts you will notice the fluid precision and rhythmic movement that results in sharpened offensive and defensive skills. Focus mitt training is dynamic and is the closest thing to replicating a sparring session. It develops precise synchronization of power, speed and accuracy.

Focus mitts, also known as target mitts, punch mitts, and punching pads are hand-held padded mitts made from dense foam covered by leather or vinyl. The mitts are held by a training partner or by a coach. The catcher (coach) and the puncher work together to create an exhilarating workout which is always engaging. The catcher gives clear and concise directions to the puncher, and the puncher responds quickly and skilfully. If an experienced coach is not available, choose a training partner with a similar skill level. Working together as a team is the key when training on focus mitts, and learning both roles is essential.

HOW THE PARTNERSHIP WORKS

Catcher Basics

The catcher must be comfortable controlling the action and setting the pace by giving instructions to their partner. Basic number sequences can be assigned for specific punches and combinations. The catcher must clearly and concisely call out punch combinations and be ready to receive the punches. The catcher calls out a number, and the puncher throws the appropriate punch. Controlling what punch is coming allows the catcher to angle the mitt properly and anticipate the force of the punch. The catcher counterbalances the force of the incoming punch by 'feeding' the mitt into each blow.

When working mitts with a partner your arm position is similar to the on-guard boxing stance, with the palms turned toward your partner ready to receive a punch. Keep your elbows slightly bent to absorb the impact of the incoming punches. Maintain stability in the body, legs, and feet staying in the classic boxing stance. Always keep your eyes on your partner and clearly communicate the combinations to be executed.

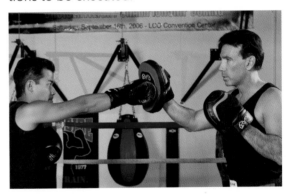

Hold the focus mitts in the correct position.

Your job is to have the mitts in the correct position to receive the punches. When catching straight punches, the mitts need to be facing forward. When catching hooks turn the palm of the mitt inward. When catching uppercuts turn the palm of the mitts downward, toward the floor. The mitts are generally held around shoulder level, but will need to be lowered slightly if training with a shorter partner or raised slightly if training with a taller partner. When two orthodox partners are working with the mitts, the left focus mitt catches the left jab and the right focus mitt catches the straight right. The same follows for hooks and uppercuts.

The catcher provides dynamic resistance by moving the focus mitts forward slightly to meet the incoming punches. This is called 'feeding' and provides the proper feel, distance, and resistance for the puncher. The receiving and resisting motion helps to reduce the impact on the catcher's shoulders. Catching punches can be a workout in itself, so be prepared by warming up the arms and shoulder regions.

Generally it is easiest to catch for someone who has the same dominant hand as you and the same boxing stance. If you are right-hand dominant, lead with your left foot forward and the left mitt ready (orthodox). If you are left-hand dominant, lead with the right foot forward and the right mitt ready (southpaw). When an orthodox catcher is working with a 'southpaw' puncher, the catcher always mimics the 'southpaw' stance with the right foot forward. The catcher stands with the right foot forward, catches the 'southpaw' jab, (the right jab), with the right mitt and catches the straight left with the left mitt. The right focus mitt catches the right hooks and uppercuts, and the left focus mitt catches the left hook and uppercuts.

Puncher Basics

Working on focus mitt drills with a partner allows you to perfect your punches while moving and responding quickly to changing circumstances. The catcher mimics the movement of an actual opponent. Unlike working on the heavy bag, the target continually moves and adjustments need to be made with your footwork, body position, and punch execution.

Start by assuming the on-guard position, ready to respond to the catcher's commands. Ensure you are the correct distance away from the catcher to throw effective punches. Stand slightly more than a jab length away from the catcher and be prepared to throw the requested punches. Stay alert and be ready to move in and out as you throw your punches. Remain on-balance, and light on your feet throwing your punches with proper technique, accuracy, and speed.

Working Together

The catcher selects the combinations and sets the pace of each round. It is crucial for the puncher to pay attention to all instructions from the catcher. Both must focus on the task, working together to create a safe training environment and developing smooth transitions between combinations. Work hard and always give your best effort.

All of our combinations are based on the puncher starting in the classic boxing stance with the left foot forward. Left jabs are thrown to the catcher's left focus mitt and the straight right punches are thrown to the catcher's right focus mitt. Left hooks are thrown to the catcher's left focus mitt. Right uppercuts are thrown to the catcher's right focus mitt.

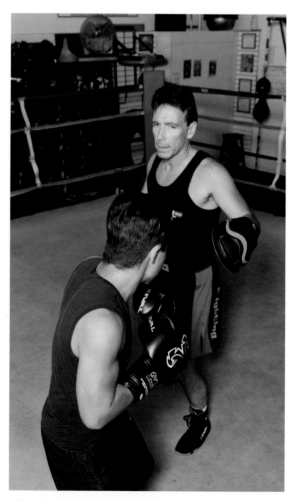

Clearly communicate the commands.

BASIC DRILLS

Building Combinations

Good communication between the catcher and the puncher is essential. Both the catcher and puncher must keep the other in view at all times. The catcher is the lead person and the puncher follows. Start with catching and receiving the basic single punches using the following number sequencing.

Assigning Numbers to Basic Combinations

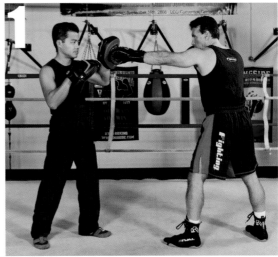

Left jab.

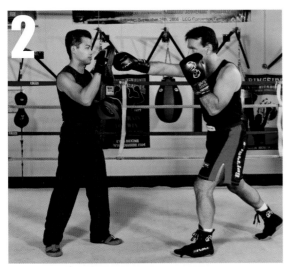

Straight right.

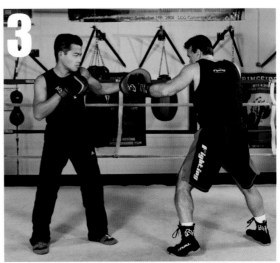

Left hook.

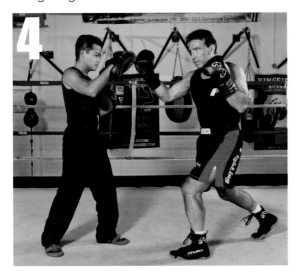

Right uppercut.

Catcher calls 1: puncher executes a left jab.

Catcher calls 2: puncher executes a straight right.

Catcher calls 1-2: puncher executes a left jab-straight right combination.

Catcher calls 1-2-3: puncher executes a left jab-straight right-left hook combination.

Catcher calls 1-2-3-4: puncher executes a left jab-straight right–left hook–right uppercut combination.

When starting to train with focus mitts, the catcher and the puncher need to practise throwing and catching the basic punches repeatedly to develop technique, reaction time, and fluidity.

'Punch and Get Out' Drill

Boxers are continually shifting between offensive and defensive manoeuvres, looking for opportunities to set up an attack and then quickly move away to a safe distance. This 'punch and get out' drill focuses on using your legs to move into proper range to deliver punches and immediately moving out of range. This 3-minute drill is broken down into 30-second intervals starting with single punch executions and gradually building a combination.

3-Minute Round Breakdown

Jab (30 seconds)

For the first 30 seconds the puncher focuses on only throwing crisp, left jabs. With the hands held high in the on-guard position move forward delivering a crisp left jab to the catcher's left focus mitt. Quickly step out and return to the on-guard position. Vary the time you spend moving around before throwing the next jab. The emphasis for the puncher is to find proper punch range, to become comfortable with balanced footwork and to maintain a good pace. The role of the catcher for this drill is to feed the focus mitt at the correct angle and to provide some resistance. The catcher allows the puncher to set the punching pace and to move around freely.

Straight Right (30 seconds)

For the next 30-second interval the puncher throws only straight rights, concentrating on moving in, landing the punch, moving out and getting ready to set up the next punch. Launch the punch by driving off the trail foot and then quickly return to the balanced boxing stance. Do not rush your punches. The foot movement portion of the drill is just as important as the punches. Work on moving in and out, and side-to-side, to develop smooth footwork.

One-Two Combination (30 seconds)

Move in toward the catcher, throw the one-two (left jab – straight right) combination and then move away. The catcher ensures that the puncher returns their hands up high to protect their face after each combination. Focus on smooth transitions from one punch to the next. The catcher must have both mitts in a ready position to receive the quick one-two.

One-Two-Three Combination (30 seconds)

This one-two-three combination (jab – straight right – left hook) starts with the puncher stepping in to land the left jab, immediately following with a straight right and finishing with a short left hook. After the left hook is landed, step away immediately and move around. Repeat the sequence. The catcher must have the mitts ready at the proper angle to receive these punches. The puncher must focus on executing crisp punches and moving smoothly.

One-Two-Three-Four Combination (30 seconds)

The puncher steps in with the left jab, followed by a straight right, then a short left hook, and finishing up with the right uppercut (jab – straight right – left hook – right uppercut). Begin by throwing light punches concentrating on the technical execution of each punch. Focus on smooth transitions from one punch to the other. As soon as you land the final punch in the sequence (right uppercut) make sure your hands are in the on-guard position. Step out, reset and repeat the sequence. The catcher must have the focus mitts in the proper position a split second before the punch makes contact with the mitt.

Four Punch Flurry (30 seconds)

For the last 30 seconds of the round throw a quick four-punch flurry, one-two, one-two (left-right, left-right) and then move out quickly. The focus is on speed, not power. Keep your punches crisp and keep your hands up.

Key Points: Basics

- After every punch sequence move out of range and get ready for your next combination.

- Ensure you are not throwing your punches with too much force as this often leads to sloppy punches and the loss of balance. Strong, efficient punches are the result of executing with proper technique.

- The main purpose of focus mitt training is to improve speed and accuracy and provide an exhilarating workout.

- When catching, feed the punches by moving the mitts slightly forward to catch the incoming punch. Keep the arms slightly bent to assist with absorption of the punch impact.

- Before moving on to the more advanced focus mitt drills ensure you are proficient with the basic combinations.

ADVANCED DRILLS

Advanced focus mitt drills allow you to mimic real fight situations in a controlled environment. These punching combinations are more complex, and slipping and ducking moves are incorporated into the drills. Intense focus is required to ensure proper execution, timing and safety.

Skilful boxers utilize defensive moves such as slipping, ducking, blocking, and parrying punches. We will be focusing on two important defensive moves, slipping and ducking in order to add a sense of realism to your workout.

Slipping

In boxing, slipping punches is an essential defensive technique. Focus mitt training is the perfect tool to master the slipping motion since the catcher is simulating throwing a punch toward you. Your previous training of visualizing punches coming at you and slipping while shadow boxing, hitting the heavy bag and double-end bag will prepare you for slipping when training with the focus mitts. Stay focused and react quickly when practising slipping combinations. Always keep the hands up in the on-guard position, bending at the waist and knees slightly and shifting the body to the left or the right to avoid the punch. Do not drop your hands and do not look at the floor. Keep your eyes on your partner at all times.

When the catcher simulates throwing a straight right or left, it is executed slowly, with minimal intent and aimed toward the puncher's shoulders, not the head region. The catcher must give the puncher sufficient time to slip out of the way.

Slipping a Left Jab: The head, body, and shoulders move as one unit to the right. Keep your body weight forward and stay off your heels, as the tendency is to lean back on the trailing foot.

Slipping a Straight Right: Dip to the left, moving your head, shoulder and body together. Always return to your balanced boxing position, hands by the face and eyes on the catcher.

Basic Slipping Combination
One-Two – Slip – Slip
The puncher starts by throwing a one-two (left jab followed by a straight right) at the catcher's mitts. The catcher immediately responds by throwing a left jab and straight right aiming for

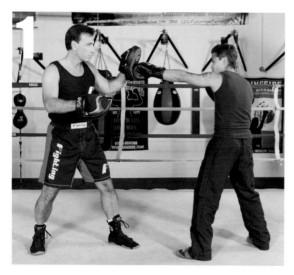

Basic Slipping Combination: Puncher throws a left jab.

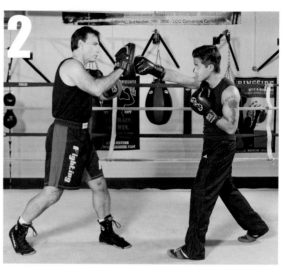

Puncher follows with a straight right.

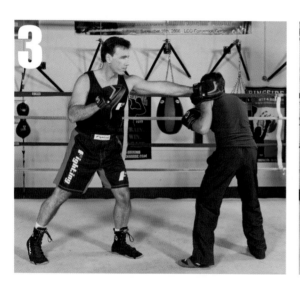

Catcher simulates a left jab, puncher slips right.

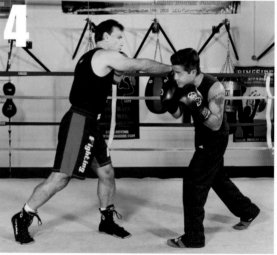

Catcher simulates a straight right, puncher slips left.

the puncher's shoulder region. The taps coming in from the catcher should be light and controlled. To avoid the incoming left punch, the puncher slips to the right and then immediately slips to the left to avoid the incoming right and left taps from the focus mitts. Develop a smooth rhythm moving side-to-side and maintaining a strong core with your hands held high.

Ducking

Boxers generally use a ducking motion to move under and avoid looping punches such as hooks. Quickly bend the knees, lowering the head and dropping the body so the punch mitt goes over the top of your head. Ducking is similar to a squat movement, bending your knees and getting down.

When the catcher simulates a left hook, the puncher dips down under the hook and over to the right to avoid the punch. When the catcher simulates a right hook, the puncher dips down and over to the left to avoid the punch. Keep your eyes on your partner. Do not bend the body forward to avoid the punch, just bend your legs. Always return to your on-guard position quickly.

To start, the catcher throws hooks slowly and high enough for the puncher to duck under. As the puncher becomes more proficient, the catcher can increase the speed of the hooks and the lower the level of the hook.

Basic Ducking Combination
One-Two - Duck - Straight Right

The puncher launches a one-two combination at the focus mitts. The catcher returns with a simulated left hook. To avoid the hook, the puncher bends both legs and ducks under the left hook, moving to the left and then follows up with a straight right. The puncher must always watch the catcher when manoeuvring under the focus mitt. The catcher needs to simulate the hook in a controlled manner allowing the puncher to duck underneath. As the timing of the punches and the ducking becomes accurate, increase the tempo of this drill.

> ### Key Points: Slipping
> - Avoid over slipping. This is when the slip is over exaggerated and you are leaning too far to the right or to the left, leaving you off-balance.
> - Keep your body weight centred through the balls of your feet. Never sit back on your heels.
> - Always keep your eyes on your partner, whether you are catching or punching.
> - A common mistake is to drop your hands out of position when you shift your body weight from side-to-side. Ensure you keep your hands up high to guard your face.

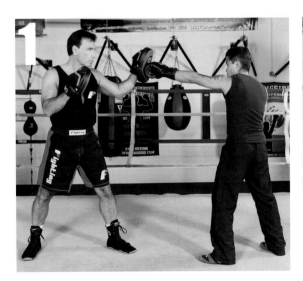

Basic Ducking Combination: Puncher throws a left jab.

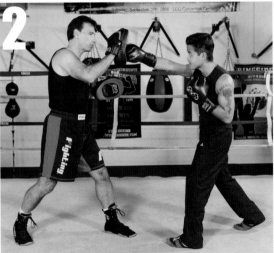

Puncher throws a straight right.

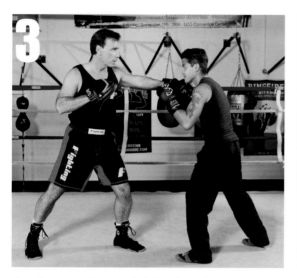

Catcher simulates a left hook and puncher starts to duck.

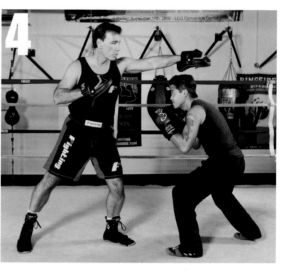

Puncher ducks under the hook.

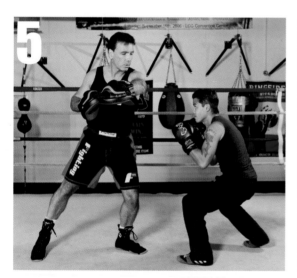

Stay balanced when ducking.

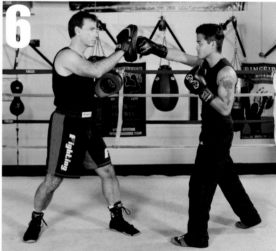

Puncher throws a straight right.

Key Points: Ducking

- Always keep looking at your partner before, during and after the combination.
- Focus on bending the legs to lower the body. Bending forward at the waist puts you off balance, puts strain on the lower back and prohibits eye contact.
- Bend your knees just enough to manoeuvre under the focus mitt.
- Practise ducking while you are shadowboxing in front of a mirror.

Building Combinations

The following six combinations and drills are broken down into easy-to-follow steps. Incorporate these combinations into your training. Remember to communicate continually with your partner while throwing and catching.

Combination 1: Jab – Jab – Right

Step 1: The puncher moves forward while executing a left jab.

Step 2: Continue stepping forward as the second jab is launched.

Step 3: Follow with a straight right from a balanced position.

(The catcher must synchronize their movement with the puncher. In this case the catcher moves backward with each punch.)

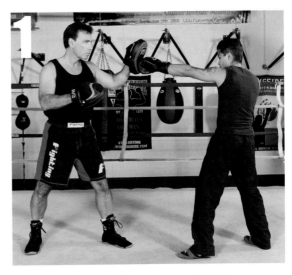

Combination 1 – Throw two quick jabs. Jab one.

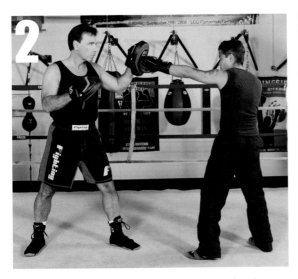

Immediately follow with another quick jab.

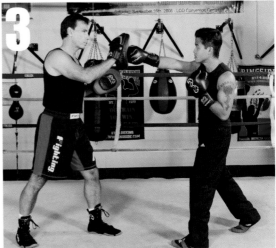

Follow with a straight right.

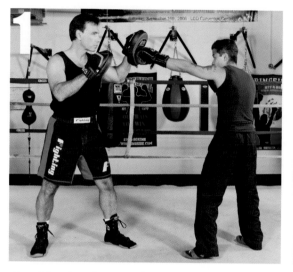

Combination 2 – Puncher throws a jab.

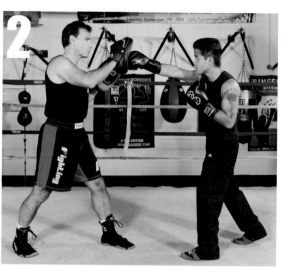

Follow with a straight right.

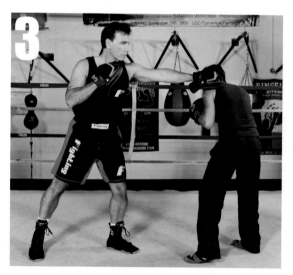

Catcher simulates a left jab and puncher slips.

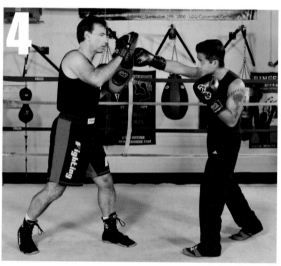

Puncher counters with a straight right.

Combination 2: One-Two – Slip – Right-Left-Right

Step 1: Puncher starts this drill with a quick one-two combination.

Step 2: Catcher simulates a left jab as the puncher slips to the right to avoid the incoming jab.

Step 3: Puncher counters with three straight punches: right-left-right.

(Remember to keep your hands up when slipping.)

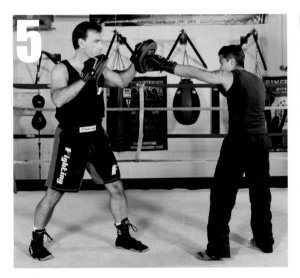

Left jab.

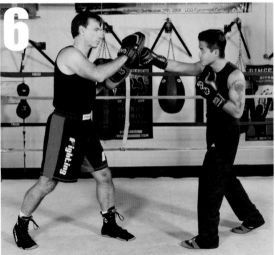

Straight right.

Combination 3: One-Two-One-Two – Slip-Slip – Left Hook – Straight Right
Step 1: Puncher throws four straight punches: left-right-left-right.

Step 2: Puncher slips the catcher's left and right mitt.

Step 3: Puncher finishes with a left hook and a straight right.

(When simulating the left and right punch, the catcher taps the puncher's left and right shoulder.)

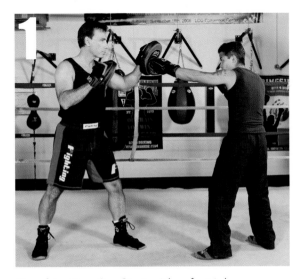

Combination 3 *– Start with a fast jab.*

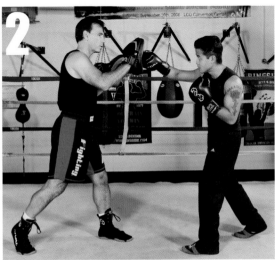

Follow with a straight right.

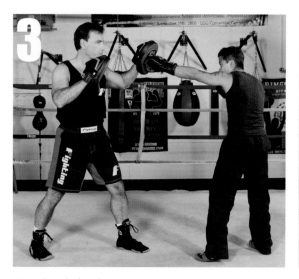

Another left jab.

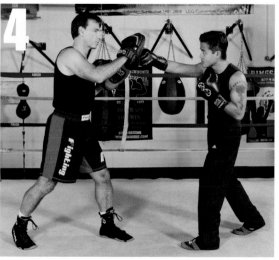

Finish with a second straight right.

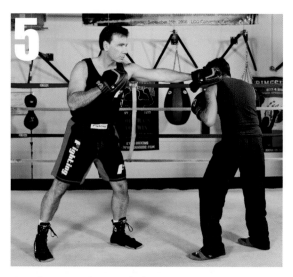

Catcher simulates a left jab and puncher slips to the right.

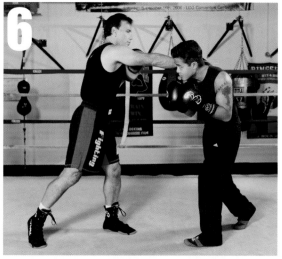

Catcher simulates a straight right and puncher slips to the left.

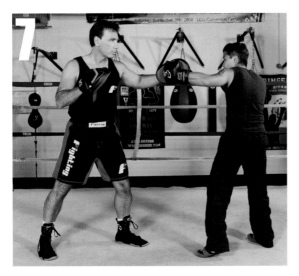

Puncher counters with a left hook.

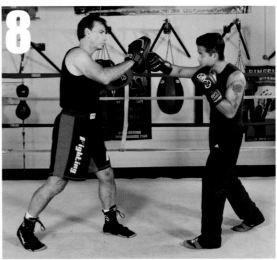

Finish the combination with a straight right.

Combination 4: Uppercut-Uppercut-Uppercut – Left Hook – Right Cross
Step 1: Catcher holds the mitts in position to receive three uppercuts.

Step 2: Puncher starts with the right uppercut first, then left, then right.

Step 3: Puncher follows with a left hook and finishes with a straight right.

(The catcher must be ready to adjust the mitts to the appropriate angle to effectively catch the punches.)

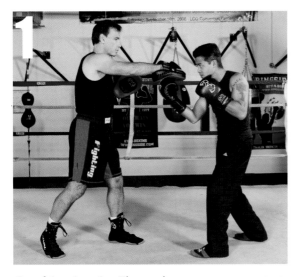

Combination 4 – *Throw three uppercuts, starting with the right.*

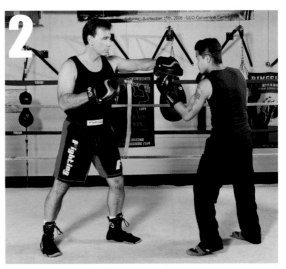

Left uppercut.

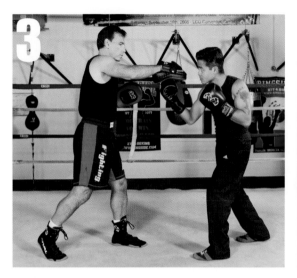

Right uppercut.

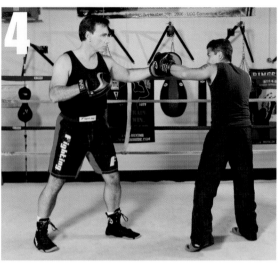

Follow with a left hook.

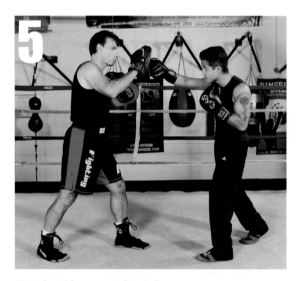

Finish with a straight right.

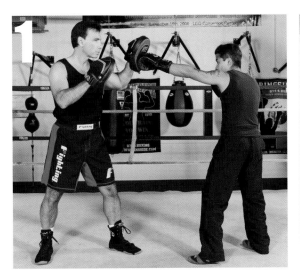

Combination 5 – Start with a sharp left jab.

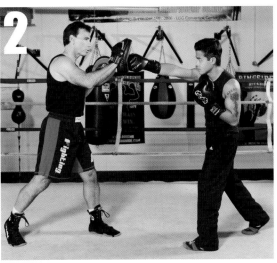

Follow with a straight right.

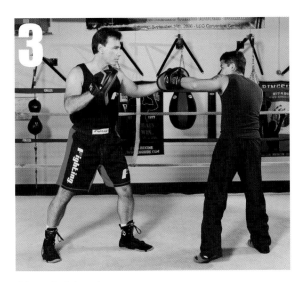

Short left hook.

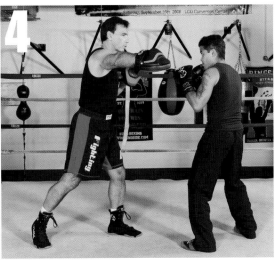

Catcher simulates a right hook, puncher ducks under.

Combination 5: One-Two-Three – Duck – Left Hook – Straight Right

Step 1: Puncher starts by throwing a three-punch combination (left jab, straight right, and left hook).

Step 2: The catcher simulates a right hook over their partner's head while the puncher ducks under the hook.

Step 3: The puncher returns with a left hook and a straight right at the mitts.

(Stay focused when ducking, body weight forward, and on the balls of your feet.)

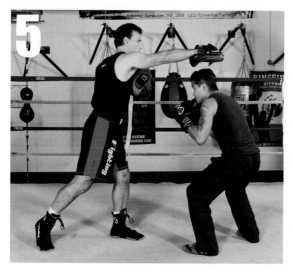

Keep your eyes on partner as you duck under.

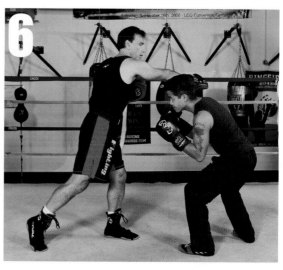

Finish with duck and prepare to throw a left hook.

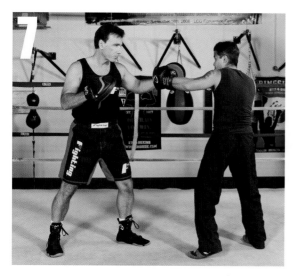

Puncher throws a left hook.

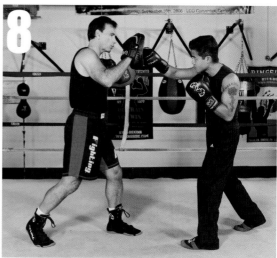

Finish with straight right.

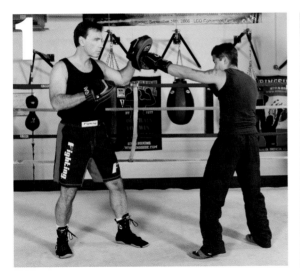

Combination 6 – Puncher throws a left jab.

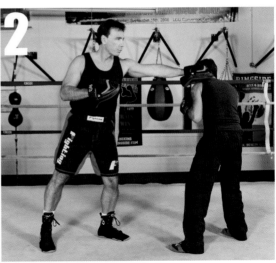

Catcher simulates a left jab, puncher slips to the right.

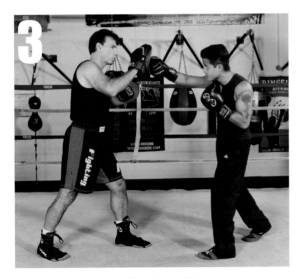

Puncher comes back with a right cross.

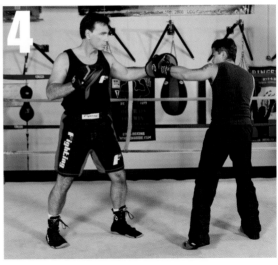

Puncher finishes with a left hook.

Combination 6: Jab – Slip – Right Cross – Left Hook

Step 1: Puncher throws a left jab to the catcher's left mitt.

Step 2: The catcher immediately comes back with a left jab, tapping the puncher on the left shoulder.

Step 3: The puncher quickly slips to the right, pivots back with a right cross and finishes off with a left hook. Be ready to move quickly.

Start by practising all of the combinations slowly and then gradually increase the pace. If you are having difficulty with any of the multiple punch sequences go back to basics combinations. Focus on crisp punches, proper technique, and balanced movement.

Creating Your Own Punch Combinations

Focus mitt training creates a dynamic training environment to sharpen skills and reflexes and to develop upper body strength. It should be challenging and fun. Work the basic combinations until you become confident with them and then add more movement and increase your punch speed. After you have perfected your skills by working on mitt drills in this chapter, start to create your own combinations. When developing your own combinations ensure they follow a logical sequence with one punch effectively setting up the next punch or movement.

It is important to modify focus mitt workouts to each individual's ability and skill level. This is accomplished by adapting the intensity level and the punch sequencing of the drills.

FOCUS MITT DRILLS

The following drills will develop your conditioning. Select one of the drills to finish your target mitt workout (a description of how to put together a complete fitness boxing training routine will be explained in Chapter 9).

Ladder Punch Drill

The puncher throws one-two combinations at the catcher's mitts and immediately drops into a push-up position on the floor and performs the same number of push-ups. Throw the left jab-straight right combination with precision each time, taking a pause to reset before you throw the next. It is not a sprint.

For example, the puncher starts in a boxing stance and throws the one-two combination eight times and then immediately drops to the floor and performs 8 push-ups. The puncher jumps up and throws 7 one-two punches and then performs 7 push-ups, then 6 one-twos and 6 push-ups and so on. Continue going down the ladder until you throw 1 final one-two punch combination and 1 push-up. (The number of punches and push-ups is reduced by one each sequence.)

For this drill the push-ups are performed with boxing gloves on. It is important to place the knuckle portion of the glove on the floor and to hold the wrists straight and steady. Both the gloves and your wraps will give additional support to your wrists. Keep the elbows close to the sides of the body, while lowering toward the floor. With more advanced push-ups keep the body long and legs straight. Beginners, start with a modified push-up with your knees on the floor. (Refer to Chapter 3 for the description of the modified push-up.) Continue to concentrate on throwing strong, straight punches at the focus mitts.

Moving quickly from a punching position down to the push-up position, and then back up to the punching position develops your agility and challenges your upper body muscles.

Depending on your fitness level, you may want to start a lower number of one-twos and push-ups. Select the appropriate starting point for you:

Basic: Start with 6 one-twos and 6 push-ups for a total of 21 push-ups/21 punches.

Intermediate: Start with 8 one-twos and 8 push-ups for a total of 36 push-ups/36 punches.

Advanced: Start with 10 one-twos and 10 push-ups for a total of 55 push-ups/55punches.

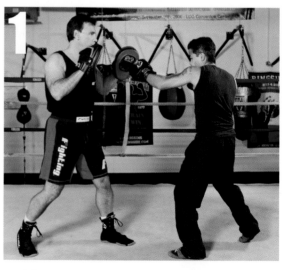

Ladder Punch Drill – Puncher throws a jab.

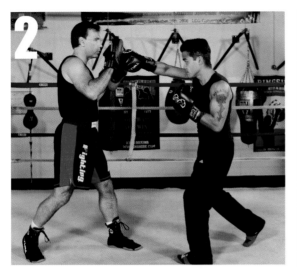

Puncher follows with a straight right.

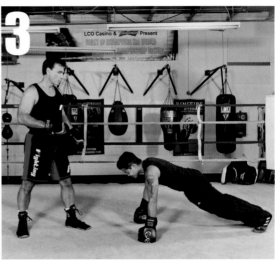

Puncher performs push-ups.

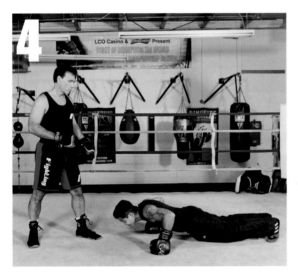

Maintain proper push-up form.

Catcher

The catcher does not stand in the traditional boxing stance to receive the punches. Instead the catcher faces the puncher straight on, holding the focus mitts at the correct angle to receive the flurry of punches. To receive the straight punches, the mitts are held facing directly at the puncher; for hooks the mitts are held with the palms facing inward; and for uppercuts the mitts are held with the palms facing downward.

For this drill, the catcher will also assist the puncher in working on slipping and ducking. At the end of the first punch sequence the catcher simulates left and right punches. The catcher throws straight lefts and rights at a consistent non-stop pace aiming at the puncher's shoulders. After the second set of punch sprints, the catcher simulates left and right hooks over the head of the puncher and the puncher practises ducking.

FOCUS MITT SPRINTS

The purpose of focus mitt sprints is to challenge and improve your endurance. This is a rapid-fire series of straight punches, hooks and uppercuts, followed by slipping and ducking moves. Focus on both speed and accuracy.

Puncher

The puncher starts this drill by facing the catcher straight on and not in the traditional boxing stance. Keeping the hands in the on-guard position and the body weight slightly forward, punch as quickly as possible. Always maintain proper punch technique. Start by throwing

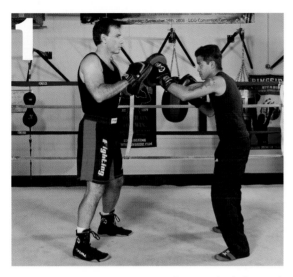

Focus Mitt Sprints - Start with straight lefts and rights.

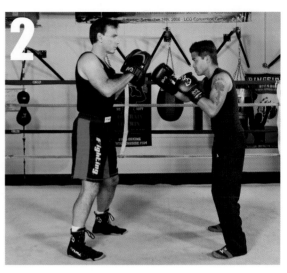

Punch as fast as possible.

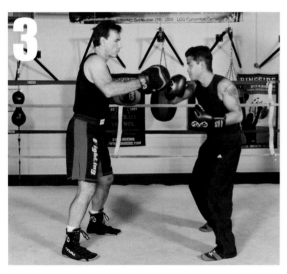

Deliver left and right hooks as fast as possible.

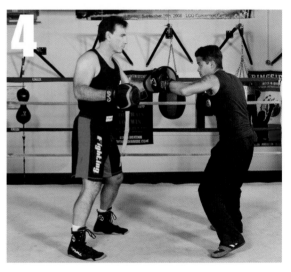

Focus on speed not power.

straight lefts and rights, fully extending your punches. Punch non-stop, starting with straight punches for the specified amount of time, moving directly into throwing hooks for the specified time and then finishing with upper-cuts. The puncher throws straight punches, hooks and uppercuts without a break. This is the first set.

Even though this is a conditioning drill and you want to maintain a swift pace, it is impera-tive that you execute the punches with proper technique. Extend your arms for the straight punches, rotate through the body when throw-ing hooks and roll your shoulders with your elbows tucked in punching up into the focus mitts for uppercuts.

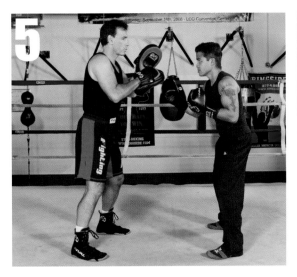

Deliver rapid-fire uppercuts.

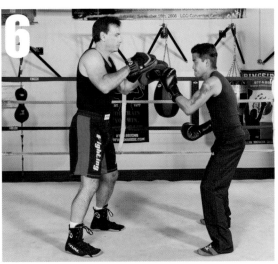

Execute technically correct uppercuts.

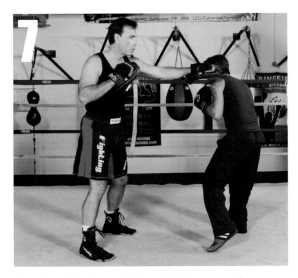

Catcher simulates left and rights, puncher slips side to side.

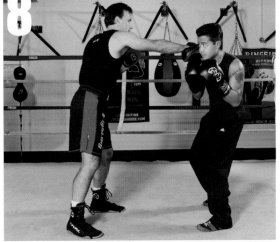

Puncher keeps hands in on-guard position and eyes on partner.

To break up the sets, slips are practised between the first and second set of punches. Slips provide a brief punching break, keeps your heart rate elevated and works your core muscles with the side-to-side movement.

The second sprint set replicates the first set, throwing lefts and right straight punches, left and right hooks, and left and right uppercuts. Ducks replace slips at the end of the sequence. When the ducking move is performed the core and leg muscles are targeted.

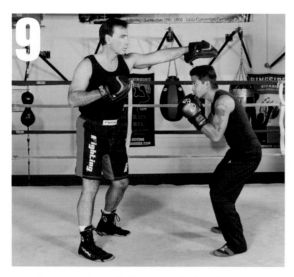

Catcher simulates left and right hooks, puncher ducks left and right.

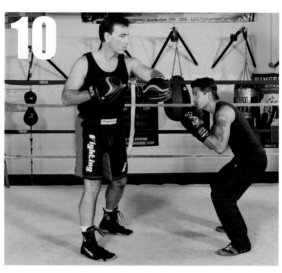

Puncher ducks under a left hook.

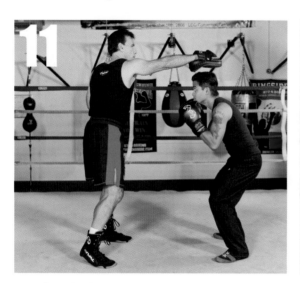

Puncher ducks under a right hook.

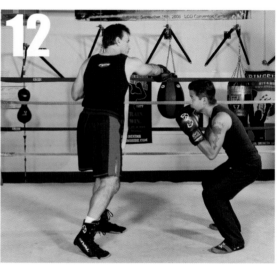

When ducking keep your body weight on the ball of your feet.

Sprint 2

Straight lefts and rights	20 seconds
Left and right hooks	20 seconds
Left and right uppercuts	20 seconds
Ducking under	20 seconds

Sample Sprint Interval

Sprint 1

Straight lefts and rights	20 seconds
Left and right hooks	20 seconds
Left and right uppercuts	20 seconds
Slipping side-to-side	20 seconds

After you have gone through the sprint sequence twice, you may want to switch roles with your training partner. Work at intervals of 20 seconds. As your fitness level improves increase the sprint time to 30–40 second intervals.

Focus Mitt Abdominal Punch-Up Drill

This 2-minute partner drill challenges your core muscle conditioning. The puncher starts in the sit-up position, lying back, knees bent and feet on the ground. The catcher stands with slightly bent knees and holding the focus mitts in proper position to catch punches.

Wearing gloves, the puncher performs a full sit-up and throws four quick straight punches (left, right, left, right) to the catcher's mitts and then returns to the ground. This is performed for a total of 20 seconds repeating the sit-ups and throwing the four quick straight punches at the top of your sit-up. Continue for another 20 seconds performing the sit-ups and throwing four quick hooks at the top of the sit-ups. For the last 20 seconds perform sit-ups and throwing uppercuts. This will take 1 minute.

Immediately repeat the sequence for another minute. The catcher must hold the mitts at the proper angle to receive each series of punches. The punches should be light with emphasis on performing smooth sit-ups. Find a comfortable pace and breathe naturally for this 2-minute drill.

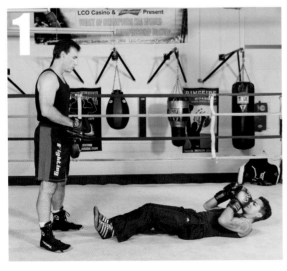

Abdominal Punch-Up Drill – Start position.

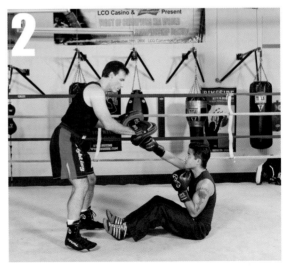

Deliver four quick, straight punches between each sit-up.

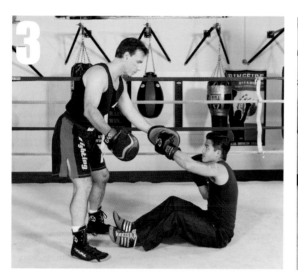

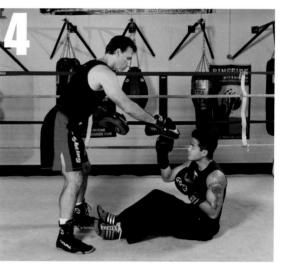

Throw four left and right hooks between each sit-up.

Throw four left and right uppercuts between each sit-up.

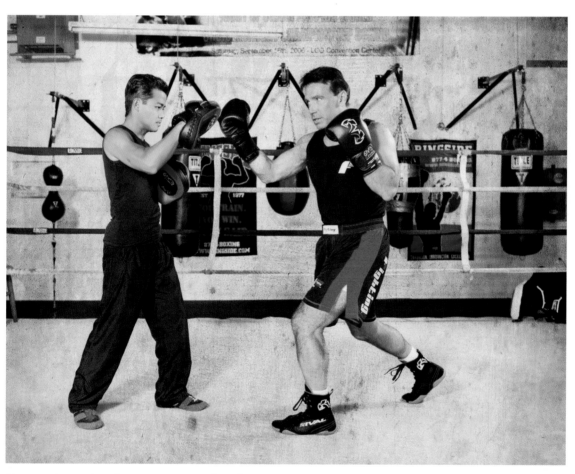

Focus mitts – develop power, speed and accuracy.

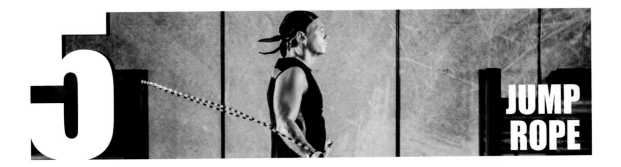

JUMP ROPE

According to the British Rope Skipping Association, 10 minutes of vigorous skipping can have the similar health benefits as a 45-minute run. (Note: the term 'skipping rope' is generally used in Britain, but 'jump rope' in North America; we use both terms here.)

Jump rope training is one of the best total body workouts and engages almost every muscle in the body. It is an effective method for improving speed, coordination and agility. It improves eye/hand/foot coordination, timing, fluidity and lateral movement. It engages the legs for jumping, the abdominals for stabilization, and uses the arms and shoulders to manoeuvre the rope.

Athletes competing in other sports like tennis, soccer, football and ice hockey recognize the benefits of jump rope training. Not only does jumping rope improve cardiovascular endurance, it will also lead to significant gains in the performance level for virtually every sport. Jump rope is not just for boxers. It is a great portable workout and you can virtually jump anywhere, indoors or outside. With practice and commitment the basic jumps can be mastered and then a wide variety of combinations can be performed.

Watch jumping footage of great boxers such as Sergio Martinez, Manny Pacquiao, Timothy Bradley, Floyd Mayweather Jr and Danny Garcia. Jump rope training is a key element not only of their leg conditioning but also their overall total body conditioning.

ROPES

Jump ropes are both practical and portable. There is an assortment of ropes available to purchase, ranging from plastic, beaded, nylon and leather ropes to weighted ropes.

A plastic beaded or segmented jump rope allows you to adjust the length of the rope and customize it specifically for your needs. Quality plastic and leather ropes allow for a fast pace and rope manoeuvrability. Nylon ropes tend to be too light, making it difficult to create a sufficient amount of momentum to produce the desired motion or arc. Weighted ropes often produce heavy, slow, awkward rotations and place additional stress on the wrists, forearms and shoulders.

The desired outcome of jumping is to develop cardiovascular fitness, fluidity and agility. A rope that is too heavy or too light defeats this purpose and may take away from your ability to concentrate on proper jumping form and technique.

Select a rope that allows for a sufficient arc and does not place additional stress on the arms and wrists. Also, choose a rope with handles that allow for easy rotation of the rope and fit comfortably into your hands.

Using a rope that is the correct length will make it easier to execute your jumps. To decide which rope length is best for you, hold the handles of the rope in each hand and stand with one foot on the middle of the rope. Pull the rope up tight. The rope handles should reach the upper chest area.

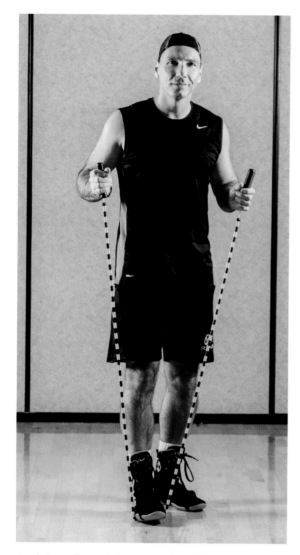

Both handles of the rope should reach chest level.

LEARNING THE ROPES

Jumping rope can be a humbling experience for even the most well-conditioned athlete. Finding a consistent, rhythmic pace comes easily for some, while others have more difficulty. Everyone has a different learning curve, and with the right attitude and motivation anyone can learn to jump rope within a few sessions. So stick with it.

Boxing follows the pattern of 3 minutes of hard work, followed by 1 minute of rest. You can choose to follow this same pattern when jumping rope: 3 minutes of jumping followed by a 1-minute rest is a great way to work up to jumping for 10-15 minutes continuously.

How to Jump

Here are some basic tips to get you started.

- Stand with your feet side-by-side, hip width apart, and your knees slightly bent.
- Hold the handles firmly (without squeezing) in your hands, with your elbows bent slightly at the sides of the body.
- The neck and shoulders stay relaxed and the head is held in a neutral position.
- Start with the rope behind your feet.
- Initiate the turning of the rope at your wrists. The shoulders and arms stay relaxed with little movement.
- Turn the rope smoothly.
- Push off the floor with both feet into the air.
- For the basic manoeuvres, your feet will only come 6-10cm (2-3in) off the floor.
- Land softly on the floor and roll through the balls of the feet to help absorb the impact.
- The torso remains upright and does not lean forward or backward.
- To reduce stress on the feet and legs, if at all possible jump on a wood sprung floor.
- Always focus on proper technique.

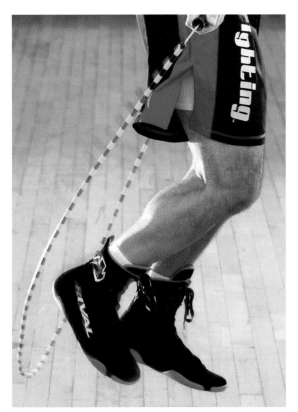

Land softly.

The Neutral Move

The neutral move is a method of swinging the rope but not jumping over it, while you concentrate on your footwork. It can help minimize the frustration of stopping and starting, and allows you to train continuously. If you are still developing your timing, it can be incorporated into your jump rope training as you try more difficult jumps or work on new foot patterns.

Place both handles in one hand and rotate the rope in a forward motion at the side of the body; ensure the rope stays at the side and does not wander in front of the body. Maintain the proper position of the shoulders, arms and wrists. Turn the rope at your wrist with the same motion as when you are actually jumping through the rope. Now you can perform the new jump sequences or foot patterns, focusing on your footwork and timing without worrying about catching the rope on your feet. Switch

the rope to the opposite hand to add variety. Once you have mastered the new jump or foot pattern hold the handles in each hand and perform the jumps through the rope.

Neutral moves, otherwise known as resting moves, can also provide a short break from jumping and allow you to continue training if you do not have the cardiovascular endurance to jump non-stop. Turn the rope at one side of the body and keep the feet moving by marching or jogging on the spot. Eventually you can reduce the amount of time using the neutral move.

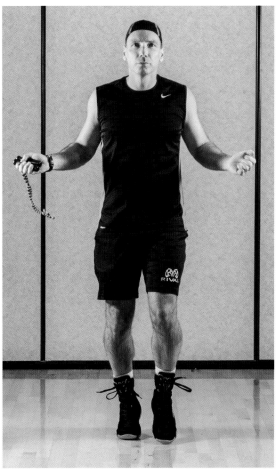

Neutral Move – Place both handles in one hand.

JUMPS

Basic, intermediate and advanced jumps are described here. With each training session you will notice that your timing has improved and you have more endurance. Continue to work on the basic jumps and then try adding some new combinations.

Basic Jumps
Basic Two-Foot Jump

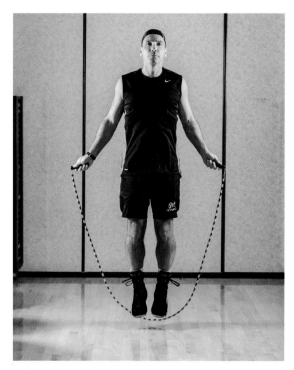

Basic two-foot jump.

The basic two-foot jump is the most common jump rope technique, also known as the 'bounce step' or 'one hop'. This is your baseline for more complex jumps and footwork. As you turn the rope keep both feet together while you jump in the air, one jump for each revolution of the rope. You will find this basic two-foot jump the easiest to master.

Start with your feet side by side and the rope behind the feet. While keeping the shoulders and neck relaxed and the head facing for-ward, push off the floor with both feet. Rotate the rope upward and over the head, then in front of the body to the floor and under your feet. Land on the balls of your feet, allowing your knees to bend slightly to absorb the landing impact. Keep the arms by the sides of the body, rotating the rope at the wrists. Aim to hold both handles at the same level from the floor. To keep the jump efficient and effective, jump fairly close to the floor, 2–4cm (1–2in). To change the intensity of this jump, increase the speed of the rope rotation.

Boxer's Skip

The boxer's skip involves slightly shifting your weight from one foot to the other with each jump. The shift in weight is subtle as both feet are still making contact with the floor. You can perform a single bounce (right foot, left foot) or a double bounce (two rights, two lefts). This is a move up from the basic two-foot jump and lays the groundwork for more difficult jumps. Relax the shoulders and neck and remember to jump just a few centimetres off of the floor.

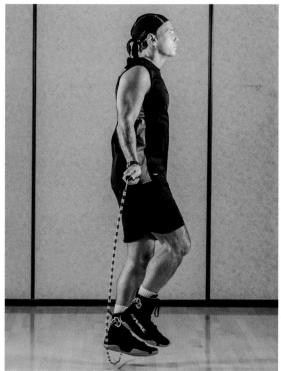

Boxer's skip – side view.

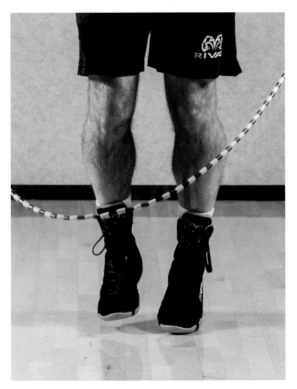

Boxer's skip – shift your weight side-to-side.

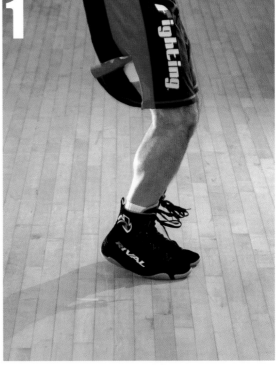

Two-foot forward and backward bounce – keep your feet together.

Two-Foot Forward and Backward Bounce

Perform the basic two-foot jump several times to set your rhythm. Keep your feet together and jump forward and then backward, travelling about 10cm (4in) when beginning. Increase your jump distance by pushing off the floor with more power. Always ensure that the natural arc of the rope is maintained.

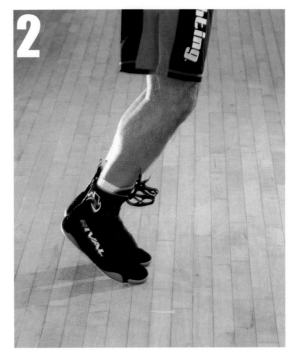

Land through your feet.

Kick-Step

Starting with the boxer's skip, lift the right foot slightly backward and then perform a small kick forward. After the kick, land on the right foot. Now lift the left foot slightly backward and kick it forward, landing on the left foot. Alternate the kicking legs and increase the difficulty by travelling forward and backward as you perform the kick-step.

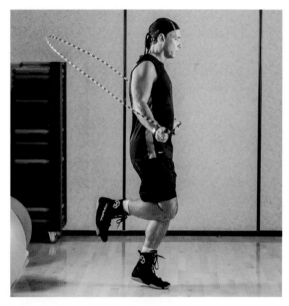

Kick-step – lift foot back.

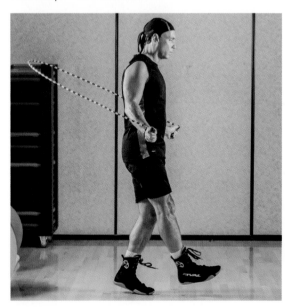

Kick-step – kick foot forward.

Intermediate Jumps
Ski Jump

For this jump begin with both feet together like the basic two-foot jump. As the rope rotates, jump to the right and then to the left, side to side, for a distance of about a 30cm (12in). A slight rope adjustment has to be made as well, since your body is moving side to side. This jump is more challenging since your feet are moving out of the centre position and the rope can easily get tangled with your feet. When performing this side-to-side jump you will find that your arms have a tendency to travel outward, so focus on keeping your elbows by the sides of the body. Try to complete four ski jumps and then go back to the basic skip. Increase the number of ski jumps as you become more proficient.

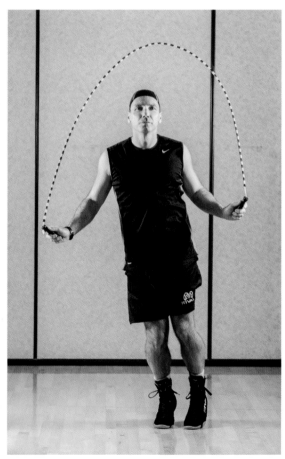

Ski jump – left.

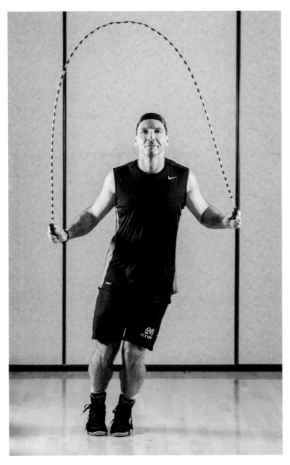

Ski jump – right.

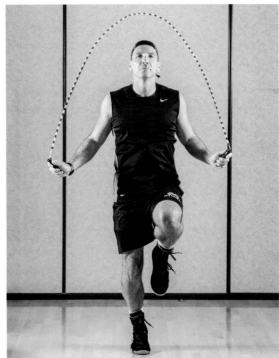

High knees – front angle.

High Knee Lifts

Similar to running on the spot, alternate lifting your knees high in front. Land softly on the floor, using the feet, knees and legs to absorb the impact. Keep the body upright and the arms in the correct position. This jump improves the muscle power in your legs. Perform 10-20 high knee lifts and then take it down to running on the spot in order to recover your breath. If you are trying to work this jump into your routine, you can add high knee lifts travelling forward and backward.

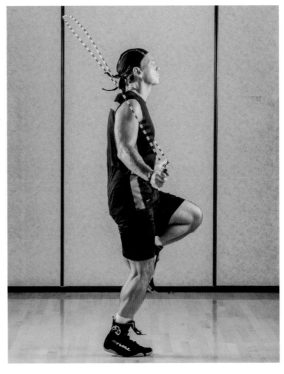

High knees – side angle.

The Ali Shuffle

During his career Muhammad Ali was known for his incredible speed, agility and quick footwork. The Ali shuffle pays tribute to the classic Ali foot movement utilized to confuse opponents. While moving around the ring Ali would suddenly shuffle his feet forward and backward, and then throw an unexpected series of punches. Practising this jump will train you to stay light on your feet and ready for any directional changes. The shifting of your foot positioning will also challenge your balance skills.

This is how to perform a slightly slower version of the shuffle. Jump in the air, moving one foot slightly forward and the other foot slightly backward, and then land on the floor with both feet at the same time. Push off the floor again, taking the front foot towards the back and the back foot towards the front. Land with both feet on the floor, alternating your feet constantly. Repeat, moving quickly and landing softly. Your agility and response time will be challenged due to the quick movement of the feet moving forward and backward.

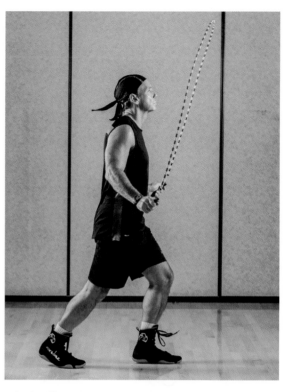

Ali shuffle – land on the balls of your feet.

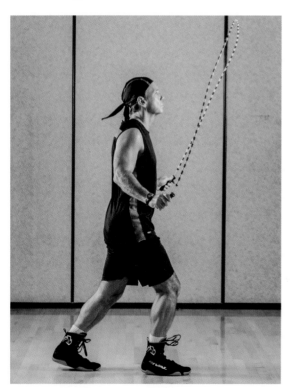

Ali shuffle – alternate your feet front and back.

Jumping Jacks

Jumping jacks are old school calisthenics and can easily be worked into your rope training. As you jump, split your feet shoulder-width apart and land softly with the feet apart; then jump again bringing the feet together and land. Repeat taking the feet apart, landing and bring the feet together and landing. When performing this jump be careful not to make the foot separation too wide as the rope will most likely get tangled with your feet. Start out with 6 repetitions and work your way up to 20.

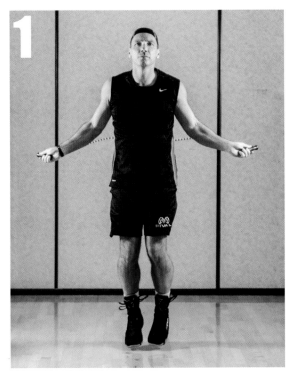

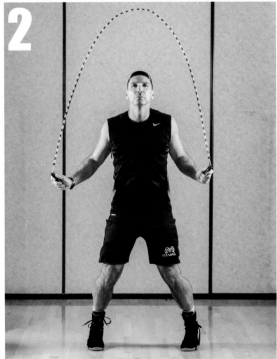

Jumping jacks – feet together.

Jumping jacks – feet apart.

Scissors

This jump has a similar foot pattern to jumping jacks but requires more timing and concentration. Perform a two-foot jump. As you jump bring the legs in, cross them in the air and land with the feet in this crossed position. Jump again, taking the feet wide and landing with a two-foot jump. Jump again bringing the other foot in front, landing in a crossed position and repeat. You may find this more challenging than the jumping jack as the crossed feet can put you off-balance. If you are having difficulty with this jump, perfect the jumping jack or practise the footwork while the holding the handles in one hand and the rope rotating at the side of the body (neutral move).

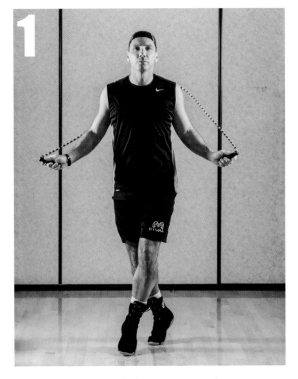

Scissors – land with feet in crossed position.

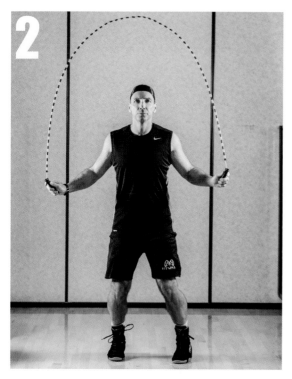

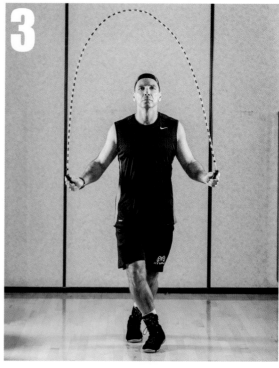

Scissors – open your feet wide.

Alternate your feet as they cross again.

Advanced Jumps
Double Unders

This demanding jump requires more leg power and increased rope speed to be successful. You must jump high enough to allow two rotations of the rope while you are in the air. The rope speed must be faster and the jump must be substantially higher than the basic jump. Double unders, also known as 'double jumps' or 'double hops', will improve your cardio-fitness and muscular endurance.

Set your rhythm by performing a few basic two-foot jumps or boxer's skips, and then perform a magnified jump with 2 fast rotations of the rope. As your timing and your fitness level improves, reduce the number of basic jumps in between your double unders. Try to perform 6 double unders, working your way up to 15.

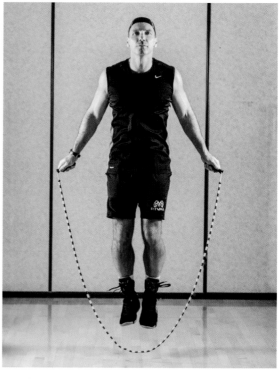

Double Unders – two rope rotations per jump.

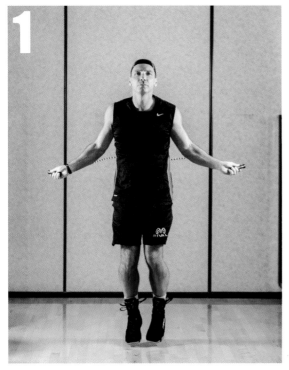

Front cross – jump high.

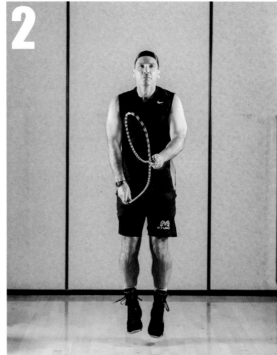

Start to cross the rope.

Front Rope-Cross

Jump at a comfortable pace. When the rope is overhead and moving forward, cross your arms at waist level and jump through the rope loop. As the rope comes overhead again uncross the arms and jump through the rope once again. When crossing the arms keep the hands by the sides of the body, with the left hand at the right hip and the right hand at the left hip. The rope handles point out to the sides and not downward.

When you perform the arm crossover motion you will have to jump slightly higher than the basic jump. Try to complete 3-4 front rope-cross jumps interspersed with a few basic or boxer's skips in between. Work up to 8-10 front rope-cross jumps in a row. This jump is also referred to as a 'crossover'.

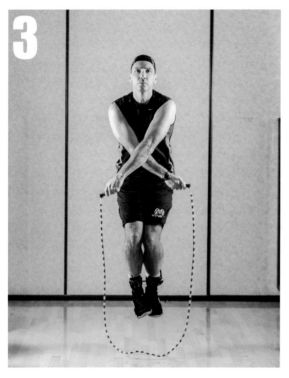

Cross the arms in front of the body.

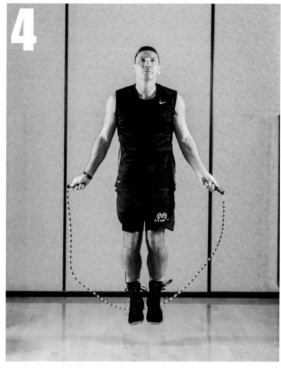

Uncross your arms.

One-Foot Jumps

One-foot jumps are basic jumps, just using one foot. If you have mastered the basic or the boxer's skip, the timing of this jump is relatively simple. The challenge comes from the demand placed on the foot, ankle and calf muscle of the working leg, and the necessity to stay on balance.

Start jumping with one foot in place several times and then switch feet. Pick up the non-working foot slightly higher, not allowing it to touch the floor. For more of a challenge add jumps from side to side or forward and backward. Start with a few repetitions working up to 8 jumps on each foot. Caution needs to be taken not to overload the leg joints and muscles when performing one-foot jumps.

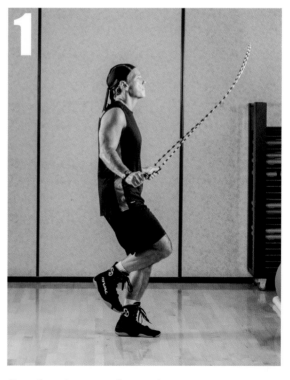

One-foot jumps – forward.

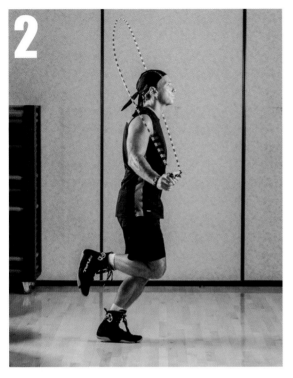

One-foot jumps – backward bouce.

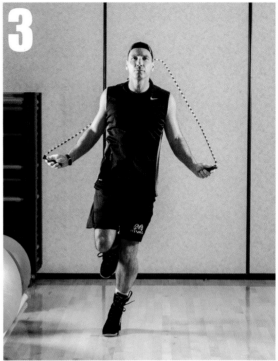

One-foot jumps – jump to one side.

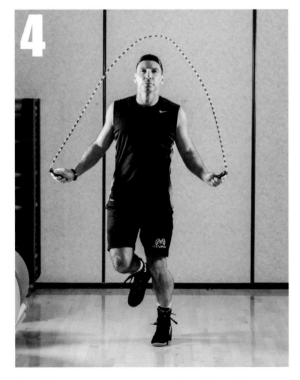

One-foot jumps – jump to the other side.

Up and Over

Lift the left knee up in front of the body, cross over the right leg to touch the floor with the left foot on the opposite side of the right foot. Lift the left knee again and touch the floor on the original start side. Repeat 8 times and then change legs. Reduce the number of repetitions down to singles with each leg, lifting the knee, crossing over to touch the floor with the foot, lifting the knee and then landing on the same foot. Keep the rope rotating smoothly, arms by the sides of the body and neck and shoulders relaxed. Always maintain an upright posture, looking straight ahead.

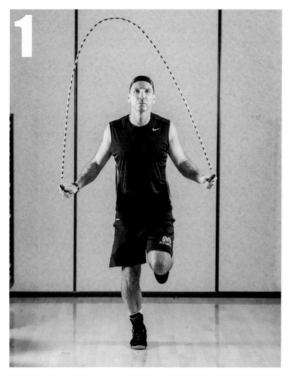

Up and over - lift one knee in front.

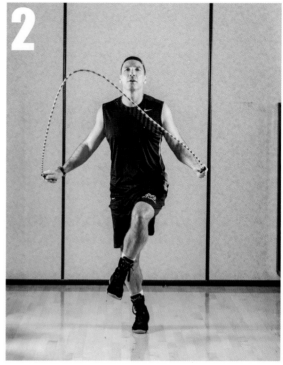

Cross the leg over.

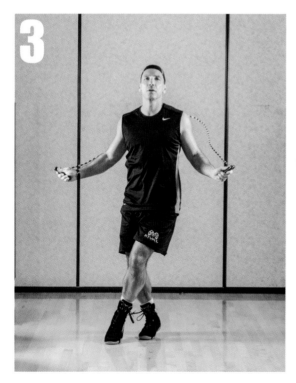

Touch in front.

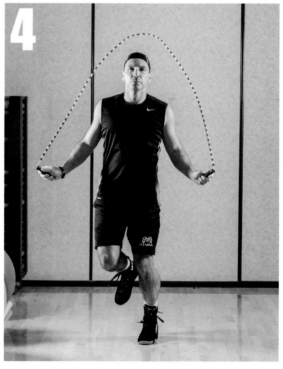

Repeat move with other leg.

Reverse Jump

Start the reverse jump with the boxer's skip, rotating the rope in a backward direction, so the rope starts in front of the feet, not behind. It is important to keep your hands and arms in the correct position by the sides of the body and not allow them to lift up and away from the sides.

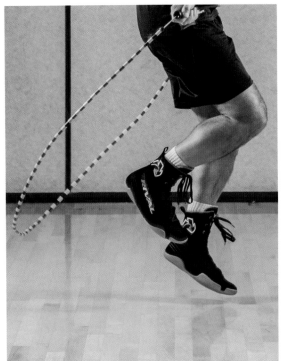

Freestyle jumping – stay light on your feet.

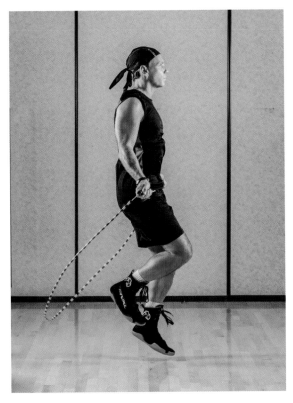

Reverse jump – rotate rope backwards.

Freestyle Jumping

Freestyle jumping keeps your workout interesting and fun by including a variety of moves. There are countless jump patterns you can perform, but to get there you need to focus on the basics. Work the fundamentals before trying more complicated jumps and then use the neutral move to develop your new combinations. Your goal is to become a freestyle jumper, incorporating a wide variety of moves and foot patterns into your skipping routine. No matter how long you decide to jump, make it fun and challenging.

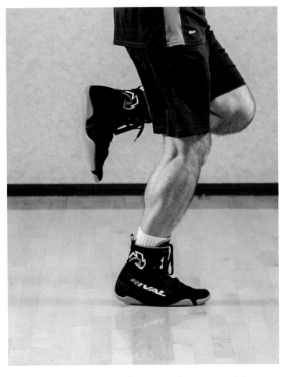

Mix up your footwork as much as possible.

Counting Your Jumps

If you are just starting out, the total number of jumps you perform is something you may want to track. Grab a rope and jump for 10-20 minutes. Increase the number of jumps you perform each workout until you build up your fitness level and your endurance. Work up to performing 2,000 jumps non-stop. This will take around 12 minutes, depending on your rope speed and experience.

JUMP ROPE DRILLS

Warm up before starting these drills, either by shadow boxing or skipping lightly for 2-3 minutes.

Jump Rope Sprints

This is an advanced, interval routine, placing demands on your shoulders, core muscles, arms and the cardiovascular system. Skip as fast as you can for short, timed intervals.

Option 1: Jump as fast as possible for 30 seconds and then rest for 30 seconds. Repeat for 10-15 sets. This drill should take you approximately 15 minutes to complete 15 sets. During the rest phase, walk around, keep moving and catch your breath. To make this drill more challenging jump as fast as possible for 30 seconds and reduce the rest time between sprints.

Option 2: Perform a 30-second sprint followed by jumping with the rope at a lower intensity for 30 seconds. Repeat for 6-10 sets.

Choose whichever jump pattern option you are comfortable with and can perform at a very fast pace. Once you become more proficient with the simple jumps try high knees or double unders all out for 30 seconds. If you miss a jump or catch the rope on your feet, keep going to keep your heart rate elevated.

Jump Rope Ladders

This interval drill helps to build your jumping stamina. Choose a number of jumps to start. For example, set a goal of 400 jumps, maintaining a consistent jumping pace. Take a 30-60 second rest. Reduce the number of jumps by 50 for each set. For your next ladder jump 350 times, then take a 30-60 second rest. Continue the down ladder to 50 jumps taking 30-60 second rests in between. During the rest periods keep moving around and when jumping keep going even if you get the rope tangled in your feet.

Jump	Rest
400	30-60 seconds
350	30-60 seconds
300	30-60 seconds
250	30-60 seconds
200	30-60 seconds
150	30-60 seconds
100	30-60 seconds
50	30-60 seconds

The total number of jumps you will perform is 1800 for the 8 sets. This should take about 14 minutes if you are resting for 30 seconds and about 18 minutes to complete assuming you are resting for a full minute. To increase difficulty, take shorter rest periods between the sets or choose a higher starting number. Initially you may want to start your ladder at 300 jumps and reduce by 50 jumps each set to the last 50 jumps.

We will show you how to incorporate jump rope into a complete fitness boxing workout in Chapter 10.

Key Points: Jump Rope

- Constantly catching the rope on your feet is often the most frustrating part for new jumpers. Ensure the rotation of the rope is moving at a constant speed.
- Perfect your foot timing by practising the basic jumps.
- Select the correct length of rope for your height.
- When turning the rope keep the arms by the sides of your body.
- Incorporate the neutral move when putting together new jump combinations.
- Move around; boxers never stay in one place.
- The speed of the rope rotations, your height, body type, fitness level and experience will influence the number of jumps performed per minute.
- A starting jumping pace is around 110–130 per minute; an intermediate jumping pace is between 130–150 per minute; and a more advanced pace is about 160–180 jumps per minute.

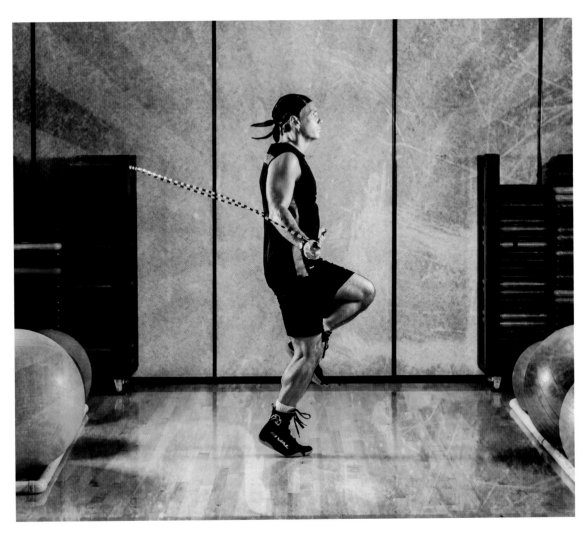

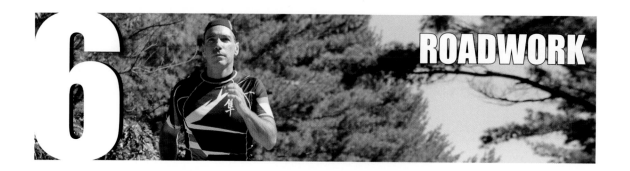

ROADWORK

From the early days of 'the sweet science', roadwork was a key element to a boxer's conditioning. Training was generally performed most days of the week and involved running for long distances at a relatively moderate pace in the early hours of the morning. The intention was to build stamina and endurance to last the entire bout and to attain the desired fighting weight. Roadwork is still a crucial part of the conditioning programme today, but the way the training is executed is very different.

Most coaches and trainers acknowledge that the sport of boxing is mainly an anaerobic sport, with approximately 70–80 per cent anaerobic demands and 20–30 per cent aerobic demands. In aerobic exercise oxygen is readily available for the working muscles over a longer period of time. Aerobic activity occurs when the boxer is moving around the ring evading an opponent, setting up an attack and catching their breath. In anaerobic exercise an activity is performed without oxygen being readily available. When boxing, the demands on the muscles and cardiovascular system are stressed at high intensities for short time periods and oxygen is not readily available. Anaerobic conditioning is necessary during a fight for the quick bursts of energy required to throw multiple punch combinations.

Today, boxers are more attentive to designing their roadwork training to mimic the demands of the sport. No longer is 100 per cent of the roadwork based on long, slow runs using the aerobic conditioning approach. Instead, when preparing for a fight higher-intensity anaerobic interval drills make up a large portion of roadwork training. Longer, medium-paced runs are often included in the training to break up the intense workouts on non-sparring days. Boxers use this more moderate approach to stay in shape between fights.

To measure how hard you really are working, whether aerobically or anaerobically, it is valuable to understand how the oxygen is pumped to the working muscles and how much effort you are putting forth.

There are a number of ways to measure the intensity level at which you are working. The assessment tool Perceived Exertion (as described in Chapter 1) is one way for you to measure how hard you are working. Monitoring your heart rate is another option for measuring your work intensity; this can be determined by counting your pulse or by wearing a heart rate monitor.

MONITORING THE HEART RATE

When your body starts to move during exercise, the heart must pump a greater volume of blood and more often, to provide sufficient oxygen to the working muscles. As the heart becomes stronger it pumps out a greater volume of blood and therefore does not need to beat as often to provide the required oxygen to the body. As you become more fit and your cardio-conditioning improves, you will notice that your heart rate decreases and beats a fewer number of times in 1 minute.

Taking Your Pulse

The pulse is a measure of your heart beating and can be used as a determination of your fitness level and how hard you are working. It is easy to find your pulse in two areas: either on

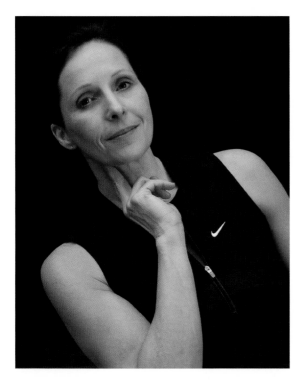

Taking your pulse – carotid artery.

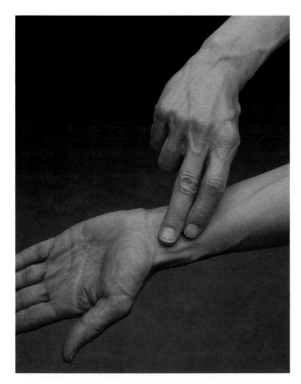

Radial artery on your wrist.

the side of the neck, just beside the trachea by placing your index finger and/or the middle finger on the carotid artery; or on the underside of the wrist by placing your index finger and middle finger on the radial artery. In order not impede the blood flow it is important that you place your fingers lightly on the arteries to feel the pulse.

Measuring your resting heart rate can be accomplished without any equipment, simply by finding your pulse while you are sitting quietly or lying down, and placing your finger on the carotid artery or radial artery. Count the number of beats in 60 seconds. This number is the amount of times your heart pumps blood to the rest of the body and can be used as a base indicator measurement. As you become more physically fit the number of beats in 1 minute will reduce because your heart becomes more efficient providing the required oxygen to the body. To measure your training heart rate while exercising, slow down your movement and place your finger on one of the arteries. Take your pulse for 10 seconds and then multiply by 6 or 3 seconds and multiply by 2 to obtain your training heart rate. The 60-second count is not generally used while exercising because the heart will slow down as soon as you slow down or stop moving.

The Training Heart Rate

As you increase your work intensity, your heart will respond by working harder and beating faster. In order to become more physically fit and better conditioned, you need to place increased demands on your heart to beat faster and work at a training heart rate level for a determined amount of time. There are a number of ways to calculate your training heart rate; we have found the most accepted and reliable method is to use the formula '220 minus your age'. This will give you your calculated maximum heart rate (MVO2). From there, a percentage rating is allocated to your predicted MVO2, depending on the intensity level you want to train.

If you are thirty years old, your calculated maximum heart rate will be 220 minus 30 (=190) beats in 60 seconds. To determine the intensity level you are training at or want to achieve, multiply the number 190 by one of the established percentages below.

Working at these different training heart rate zones provides specific results. If you want to work at a steady rate for a sufficient amount of time (endurance training), multiply 190 by 60 per cent and 70 per cent (190 × 0.60 and 0.70) to give you a training heart rate of 114–133 beats in 60 seconds or 19–22 beats in 10 seconds. Take your pulse at the carotid artery or radial artery site to obtain the number of times your heart beats in 60 seconds or 10 seconds. Once established, either increase your exercise effort or decrease it in order to match up with the desired training heart rate zone.

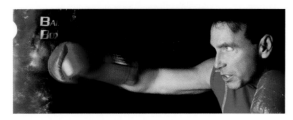

Vary your training intensity.

Training Heart Rate Zones

Endurance Conditioning (60–70 per cent)

Training at a moderate rate, developing both cardiovascular and muscular efficiency. Your heart rate increases somewhat, and you will breathe slightly faster. Fat is mostly used as the energy source. This is equivalent to the 4–5 rating on the Perceived Exertion Scale.

Aerobic Conditioning (70–80 per cent):

The training intensity is taken up a notch. Your breathing rate will increase, talking becomes more difficult and you start to sweat. Training at this slightly higher rate assists in improved cardiovascular conditioning, muscular strength and weight control. The fuel source is both fat and carbohydrates. This is equivalent to the 6–7 rating on the Perceived Exertion Scale.

Anaerobic Conditioning (80–90 per cent):

You are training hard, breathing becomes strenuous, it becomes difficult to talk and your muscles fatigue quickly. This is the level you will be working at when performing intervals or speed work. Training at this level improves your lung capacity and enhance lactate tolerance. This is equivalent to the 8–9 rating on the Perceived Exertion Scale.

VO2 Max (90–100 per cent):

Training at your limit. You will only be able to sustain this intensity for a very small amount of time, most likely less than 1 minute, and you will not be able to talk. Training at this level will enhance your speed and efficiency. This is equivalent to the 10 rating on the Perceived Exertion Scale.

Remember to train at the intensity level specific to your desired outcome and specific to the demand of the exercise you are performing.

Heart Rate Efficiency

The length of time it takes for your pulse to return back to your resting heart rate is a great indicator of your fitness level. As you become increasingly more physically fit, the faster your heart rate will recover back to your resting heart rate after a workout. Also over a period of training weeks, your trained heart becomes stronger and supplies a greater amount of blood to the working muscles with less effort and has to therefore, beat less often. You will be able to perform at a higher level with less effort.

Heart Rate Monitors

An alternative to taking your pulse manually is to use a heart rate monitor to help you determine how hard you are working. There are many types of heart rate monitors available which offer you real-time data while you are training. The basic models record your heart rate at rest and during your training. Also, many heart rate monitors can be pre-programmed to assist training at different workout levels.

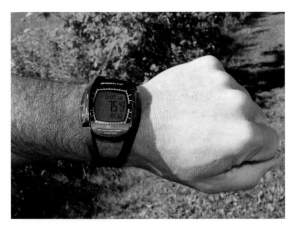

Heart rate monitor.

An electrode, usually on a band, is positioned either around the chest or the arm and will detect your working heart rate. This information shows up on the corresponding watch, allowing you to monitor your intensity level without stopping or slowing down to locate your pulse. Excessive motion and moisture, however, may produce imprecise readings.

Some other features many heart rate monitors include are:

- Time in target zone: This feature monitors the amount of time you spend exercising within your desired target heart rate zone. Depending on the objective of your training, ideal training times will vary.
- Recovery heart rate mode: This records the time it takes for your heart to return to its normal resting rate, useful for monitoring sprint and interval workouts. You can also use this to evaluate your cardiovascular fitness, reviewing the length of time it takes for your working heart to return to a resting rate.
- Speed and distance monitor: The speed and distance of your run is measured for a specific workout. Generally a GPS receiver is used for outdoor workouts and a foot pod, measuring stride length, is used for indoor workouts.
- PC interface: This feature allows you to connect the information from the heart rate monitor to your computer, allowing training statistical analysis and storage.

The heart rate monitor is a useful tool for you to understand how your heart reacts to exercising and is a guide to access your cardiovascular fitness over a period of time. It does not, however, take into account other physiological or psychological factors that can influence your training intensity. Many factors will influence your heart rate, such as stress levels, your health status, the environmental temperature whether very hot or cold, when your last meal was digested and the natural rhythms of your body. Always pay attention to your running intensity – how hard or easy it feels – and employ the perceived exertion rating scale as a resource.

TIPS FOR EFFECTIVE RUNNING

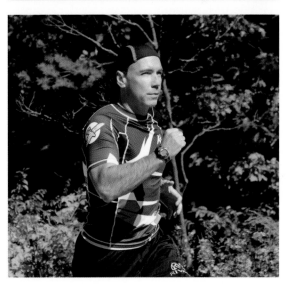

Effective running technique.

Body Position

Head Tilt
Posture is extremely important when running and assists in your running efficiency. Look straight ahead in front of you; do not look down at your feet. This will help you to maintain a straight neck and back, and your chin in a neutral position.

Shoulders
Keep the shoulders low and relaxed throughout your run. As you become tired the tendency is to raise the shoulders up toward the ears and often dip side to side with each foot strike. Relaxed shoulders also play an important role in maintaining the proper posture for efficient running.

Arms
Swing your arms straight forward and backward in combination with your leg strides. Keep your elbows at a 90-degree angle for the most part. If you feel your arms, hands and neck region tensing up, drop your arms to your sides and shake them out. Ensure your hands are relaxed in an unclenched fist.

Torso
The torso is held upright with the core muscles held taut, with your head up looking forward and your shoulders relaxed. Running in this tall position assists with optimal breathing and proper stride length.

Hips
Your hips are key to good running posture. When the torso and back are straight and upright the hips will fall into the correct alignment. Keep the hips in a neutral position, avoiding an extreme tilt forward or backward.

Knees
The knee position establishes your stride length. Seasoned endurance runners lift their knees only slightly giving them a quick leg turnover and a shorter stride. This allows for an efficient forward movement that wastes very little energy.

When sprinting, the knees are lifted higher in order to produce maximum leg power. The knees move straight forward as you lift them and directly below the hips as you land. When your foot strikes the ground a slightly bent knee will absorb some of the impact.

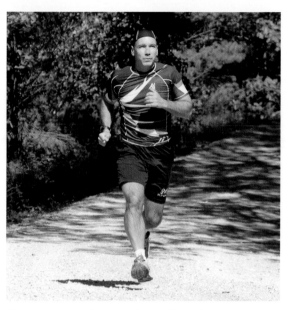

Keep neck and shoulders relaxed.

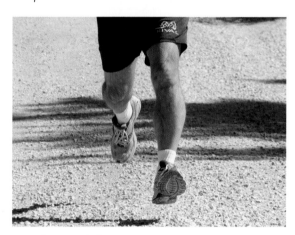

Aim for quick foot turnover.

Feet
Proper foot placement and push-off will help you to run well. Land with your foot lightly on the ground between your heel and mid-foot, and roll quickly toward the toes. Push off the front of your foot, getting extra power from your ankle and calf muscle. Keep the contact time of the foot with the ground to a minimum. The aim is to achieve a quick turnover time.

Warm up Before you Run

It is important to warm up before starting any running program. A great way to increase the blood flow in your body is to warm up by shadow boxing, moving side-to-side and forward and backward, throwing punches. You can also warm up by walking for 5 minutes at a fairly good pace, swinging the arms and stretching out the muscles if they feel tight. Perform pre-activity stretches (see Chapter 8).

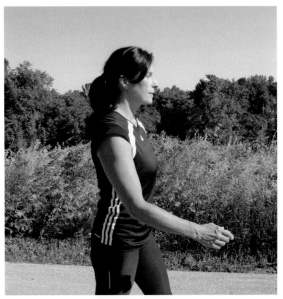

Walk/run method-start by walking.

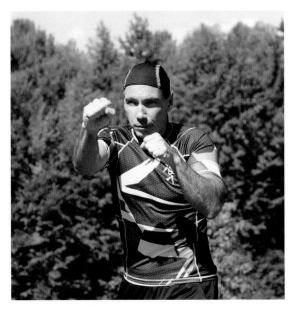

Warm-up by shadowboxing.

A RUNNING PLAN

How to Start Running

If you are new to running, a safe approach is to walk and run in intervals. You will build stamina to run further and faster and not place your joints and muscles at risk of injury. This slow and steady method of training starts with walking for a specific time or distance, followed by jogging for a specific time or distance. When beginning a running program take 24 to 48 hours in between your training. It is during these non-training rest days that the body mends and your fitness and strength improves.

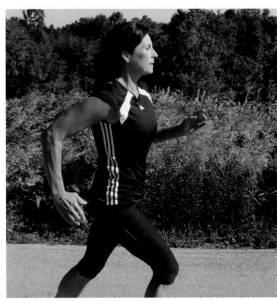

Walk/run method-run.

Depending on your base level of fitness, start by walking (2-5 minutes) and jogging (2-5 minutes), intermittently for a total of 12-15 minutes.

Then decrease the amount of time you spend walking and increase the amount of time you spend running. Work at a moderate to hard perceived exertion rate of 6-8. Your breathing will increase and you will start to sweat. During the walking phase, walk fast and keep the heart rate elevated, still working at a moderate level. The first three to four weeks are generally the most difficult for novice runners. The body and musculature is adapting to the new demands placed on it. Listen to your body and monitor your running/walking time and intensity. You do not want to get into an intense training situation where you are gasping for air or placing too much stress on your muscles and joints.

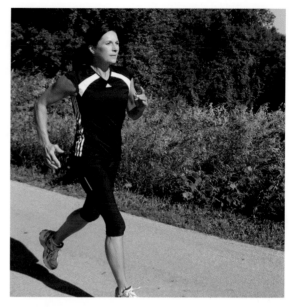

Build your stamina.

Key Points: Running Basic

- Look straight forward, keeping your neck and back straight and your chin in a neutral position.
- Move your arms forward and backward beside the torso with each foot strike.
- Listen to your body and work up to running a continuous distance.
- Land your foot softly on the ground and let your knee and ankle absorb the impact.
- Maintaining a tall posture will assist with your breathing.
- Stop and stretch out your muscles if they become tight during a longer run.

Building Cardiovascular Endurance

If you are able to run for 15-20 minutes comfortably, continue to increase the distance and time spent running. Make the increases every two to three weeks aiming for a continuous running/jogging for 45-60 minutes. Run at a moderate perceived exertion rate of 6-7.

Remember to stretch out the muscles and joints after these longer runs, especially the hip flexors and calf muscles (see Chapter 8).

RUN LIKE A BOXER

All types of cardio-training are important for boxing. To fight effectively a boxer needs to train to maintain their strength and endurance, but they also must be able to produce intermittent explosive bursts throughout every round.

A weekly running programme consists of intervals, sprints and an occasional aerobic longer run. The longer runs help to maintain and improve cardio-respiratory endurance to last the length of a boxing match. Interval training develops the conditioning required to sustain a higher effort level for a specific time or distance. Sprints prepare the body for an all-out effort.

Interval Training

To improve your running performance, you need a balance of easy running and the more difficult, faster intervals. Relating back to the 'overload principle', additional stress is a requirement for improved performance. Interval running sessions provide the added stress so your fitness level can adapt and evolve, and not stay at a stagnant level. Work at a perceived exertion of 6-7 for the basic running and then bump up the intensity to 8-9 for your interval running for a specified distance or time.

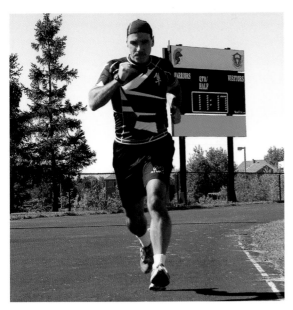
Interval training track sprints.

Sample Routine
Start with a warm-up (jogging for 1km). Perform your interval training by running at a perceived exertion of 8-9 for 2 minutes or 400m. Reduce the intensity to 6-7 for 1 minute. Repeat these higher intensity intervals six times, with a 1-minute lower intensity run in between. Finish off with an easy 1-2 kilometre jog.

Interval Training With Sprints
Including interval training with sprints in your workout helps to push you beyond a fitness plateau, thereby improving your physical conditioning level. Sprints challenge your heart strength and endurance, and your muscle capabilities. To perform a sprint, an all-out effort is required for 10-30 seconds or running a distance of approximately 200m. Work at a perceived exertion of 10. At this level it will be difficult to keep up this pace.

Distance Sprints
A basic form of interval sprint training is to sprint the same distance repeatedly. This can be easily measured if you perform the sprints on a track. Always start by warming up your muscles and cardio system by jogging for 400m. Now sprint (perceived exertion level of 10) for the same distance repeatedly; for example 200m. Keep up this running intensity for the 200m distance and then jog or walk back to your starting point. Use the time it takes to jog or walk back to the start location to recover. When sprinting breathe deep into your abdomen, pump your arms and lift the knees high. Repeat six times, and cool down with an easy jog.

Timed Sprints
Timed sprints require you to run at a perceived exertion level of 10, for 30 seconds. Always warm up with a 6-10 minute jog and start your sprint by steadily increasing your speed to maximum. Try to recover within 1 minute by walking or jogging and then perform another all out 30-second sprint. Perform 30-second sprints six times with a 1-minute rest in between. Access your consistency by tracking the distance you travelled in the 30 seconds. Finish off with a 6-10 minute easy run.

Interval Hill Sprints
Running up hills is a great way to challenge your overall conditioning and work at a higher intensity level without placing excessive impact on your joints. The inclined surface increases the difficulty of the run. If you are running outdoors plan a route that includes hills.

When sprinting up the hill, lean slightly into the hill, keeping your chest up. You will notice that your stride is shorter and you will have to lift your knees higher. It is best to shift your foot plant to the balls of your feet. Keep the arms and legs working in unison, pushing forward as you approach the top. Try to run past the top and then relax as you run or walk down the hill, allowing gravity to help pull you along and allowing your stride to open up. Always focus on proper running technique. Warm up by running for 8-10 minutes and then sprint up a hill at a perceived exertion of 9-10 for 30-60 seconds. Walk or jog down the hill to recover. Repeat six to eight times.

Interval running or sprinting sessions can be performed 2-3 days per week but never on consecutive days. Since these workouts are intense, your body requires adequate time to recover. It is also advisable not to perform sprint intervals on the days that you train on the bags and focus mitts.

An additional benefit of training at this very high intensity is that more energy is required and therefore more calories are burned. If one of your goals is to lose weight, then incorporate sprints into your training.

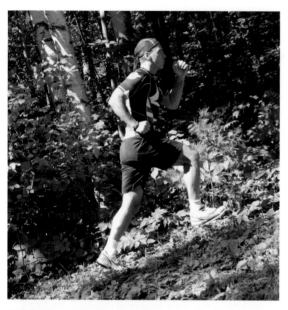

Hill Sprints – challenges your overall conditioning.

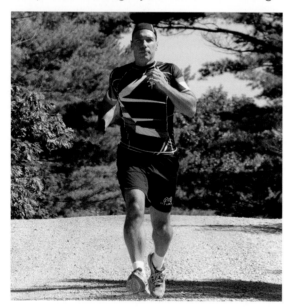

Downhill technique – allow your stride to open up.

> ### Key Points: Sprints
> - Start your foot turnover at a moderate pace, gradually increasing to your maximum sprint speed.
> - Adjust or lessen your pace if you feel pain or distress.
> - Always warm up your muscles, joints and cardiovascular system before performing sprints.

TREADMILL ALTERNATIVE

If you are unable to run outside due to the weather or the location, then running on a treadmill is a great alternative. Simply walk or run in place keeping up with the motorized belt that moves under your feet. The newer models provide sufficient shock absorption, a wide variety of training programs and storage for your personal programs.

Start with the treadmill moving slowly, placing one foot on either side of the belt. Step onto the moving belt. Do not hold onto the handrails unless you are very new to working on the treadmill. Move your arms when running on the treadmill as you would when running outside. If however you are experiencing any balance issues, then steady yourself by lightly touching the handrails. Maintain an upright posture and look straight ahead.

Running on the treadmill burns approximately the same number of calories as running outside. There is a difference though, when running on an inclined treadmill compared to running up hills: running up hills takes more energy and burns more calories than running on an inclined treadmill.

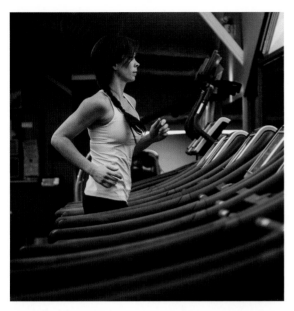

Cardio alternatives – treadmills are a good option.

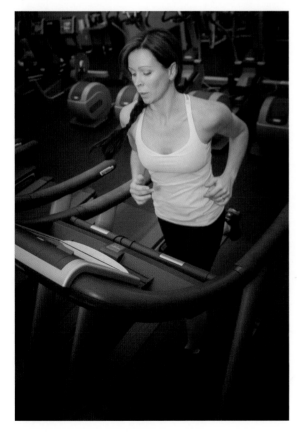

Treadmill can be programmed for interval workouts.

CLOTHING

Footwear

Choose running shoes that provide good heel support, have mid-sole flexibility and adequate sole cushioning for your weight. Go to a reputable sports store with knowledgeable and trained staff, and try on running shoes that are designed for your running style.

Warm Weather Running

When running in hot weather it is ideal to wear light coloured, loose-fitting clothing made from breathable fabrics. Wear sunglasses or a visor to protect your eyes from the sun, and always wear sunscreen on any exposed skin. Avoid training in the hottest part of the day. It is often best to run early in the morning or later in the day after the sun has set, staying away from the direct sunlight. Reduce your exercise training intensity level, as your heart rate may increase because of the heat. Stay hydrated by drinking water before, during and after your run.

Cold Weather Running

When running in cold weather layer your clothes. Wear clothing with moisture transport qualities close to your body and a breathable windproof jacket and pants over the top. To prevent the loss of your body's heat through your head, wear a toque or balaclava. Keep your hands warm by wearing gloves or mitts, and if the sun is shining, remember to wear sunscreen and sunglasses for protection especially against the glare of snow on the ground. It is best to avoid training outside if the temperature drops below 10°C (15°F), or in extremely windy or icy conditions. Be aware of the surface you are running on and if it is slippery shorten your stride length to improve your footing.

Performing roadwork within your training schedule will improve your cardiovascular fitness and is included in the Fitness Boxing workouts in Chapter 10.

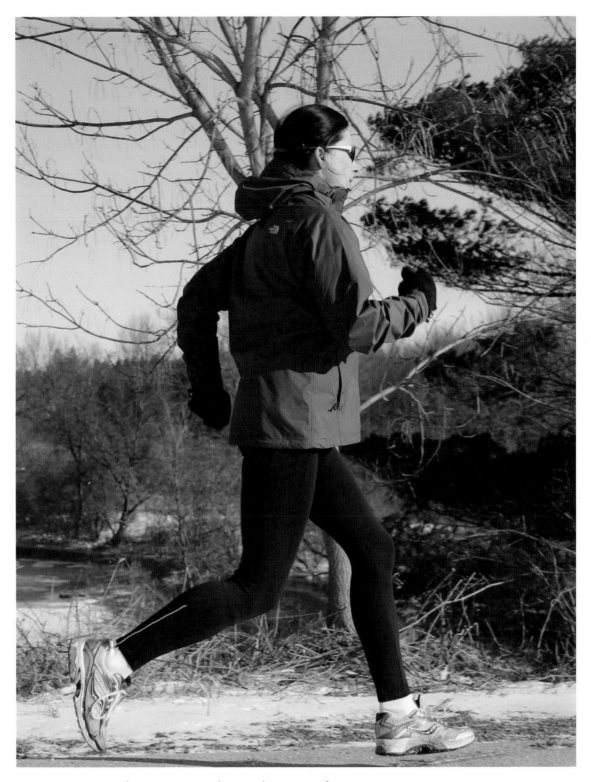

Winter running – shorten your strides on slippery surfaces.

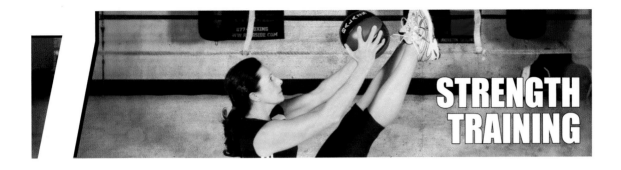

The origins of boxing can be traced back to ancient Greece and Rome. Those brutal matches, though, hardly resemble the intricate physical science that boxing has become today. The medicine ball also has an ancient history. It was nearly 3,000 years ago that the Greek physician, Hippocrates had his patients toss primitive sand-filled sacks around to develop musculature for injury prevention and rehabilitation. Persian wrestlers trained using their version of a medicine ball to build strength and stamina to get ready for a match. The medicine ball is still used today and has evolved over many centuries.

As strength training evolved for boxing, exercises were designed to condition the abdominal muscles. One old-school exercise was to simulate body punches by tossing a leather medicine ball to the abdominal region of the boxer. It was thought that this type of drill would develop stronger abdominal muscles to absorb the body punches. Thankfully today there are many more effective exercises that do not involve throwing a ball to somebody's mid-section.

The medicine ball delivers an incredibly dynamic, effective workout for core muscle development and upper body and lower conditioning. The ball can be lifted, pushed, pressed, thrown or tossed. Medicine ball training challenges reaction time, alertness and agility. Compared to working with just weights the exercises with the medicine ball allow for a greater range of motion at the joint areas and involve more muscles and movement. It is one of the most versatile strength training tools.

MEDICINE BALL BASICS

The Ball

Traditionally the medicine ball was made from leather but is now available with such materials as rubber, vinyl and neoprene for the outer covering. The balls are filled with materials such as sand, steel shot and gel-filled polyvinyl chloride shells. The weights range from 1kg to 14kg (2–30 lbs). Choose a medicine ball weight that allows you to complete 8 to 14 repetitions of the exercise and 2 to 3 sets. When the exercise calls for the ball to be placed on the floor, a larger sized ball will offer a more stable base and is a better choice.

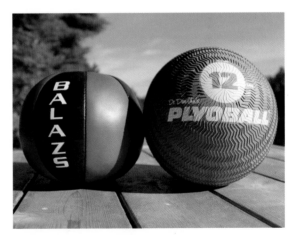

Modern medicine balls.

Keep a Grip

Keep your core tight as you execute the moves, maintaining proper muscle alignment. Ensure you have a firm grip on the ball. When working with the medicine ball all movement should be smooth and controlled.

Breathing

Remember to exhale on exertion, when you press or push the medicine ball away from your body. Inhale when returning the ball back to the starting position or in the relaxation phase of the exercise.

Which Exercise Level?

The medicine ball exercises are rated as basic, intermediate and advanced. Select the appropriate exercises for your fitness level.

UPPER BODY EXERCISES

Standing Medicine Ball Twist (Basic-Intermediate)

Targeted area: Deltoids, obliques, abdominus recti, latissimus dorsi, trapezius.

Hold the medicine ball in front of the body at shoulder level with the arms fully extended. Keep the arms extended as you rotate your body as far as you can to one side. Then rotate toward the other side. This is one repetition. The shoulder muscles fatigue first, so choose a medicine ball at a lighter weight. For added intensity rotate to the side further and swivel onto the ball of the opposite foot.

Suggested repetitions and weight: Perform 1 to 3 sets of 8 to 12 repetitions with a 3-5kg (6-10lb) medicine ball.

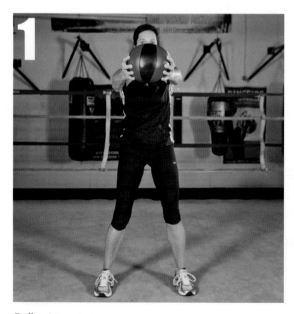

Ball twist – start.

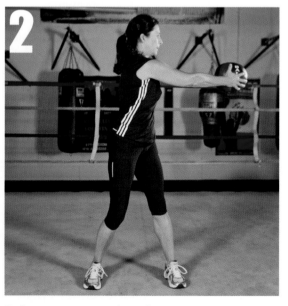

Ball twist – rotate to the side.

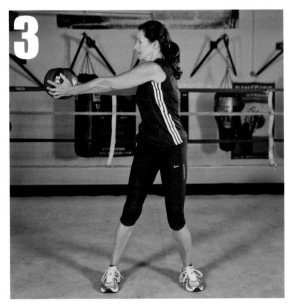

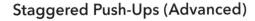

Ball twist – rotate to the opposite side.

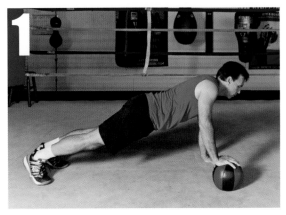

Staggered push-up – up position.

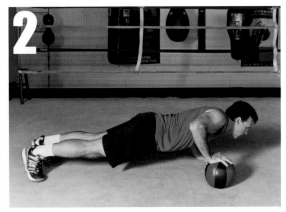

Staggered push-up – down position.

Staggered Push-Ups (Advanced)

Targeted area: pectoralis major, serratus anterior, triceps.

These push-ups are challenging because the ball provides an unstable surface. With one hand on the ball and the other on the floor, obtain a push-up position. The muscles of the shoulders and the rotator cuff are required to stabilize the torso as the push-up is being executed. Ensure you perform the push-ups in a slow and controlled manner, exhaling on exertion when you push-up and inhaling as you lower your body.

If you are just starting out reduce the stress on the shoulders by modifying the push-up and placing both knees on the floor. Select a medicine ball that is larger in size to give you a more stable base.

Suggested repetitions: Perform the push-ups on one side, then switch the ball to the other hand and repeat. Perform 2 sets of 10 to 12 repetitions.

The Boxer's Push-Up (Advanced)

Targeted area: pectoralis major, serratus anterior, triceps.

This advanced push-up requires extra strength and control through the core, arms and shoulders to maintain perfect balance. Both hands are placed on the medicine ball and the body is in the push-up position. Maintain a strong body with the abdominals held tight and the hands held close together. Lower the body towards the ground keeping the elbows pointing back and inhale; then raise the body and exhale.

Once again, execute the push-ups from both knees if you are having difficulty maintaining a strong core. Select a medicine ball that is larger in size to give you a more stable base.

Suggested repetitions: Perform 2 to 3 sets of 8 to 12 repetitions.

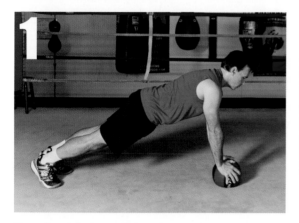

Boxer's push-up – start.

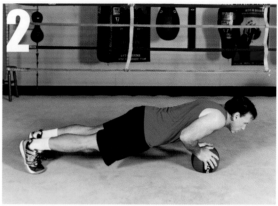

Stay balanced as you lower your body.

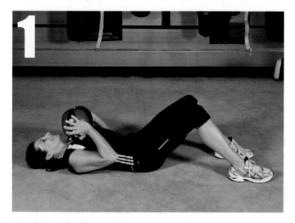

Medicine ball crunch – start position.

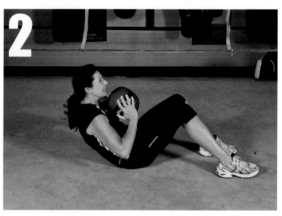

Lift your head and shoulders in a smooth motion.

CORE STRENGTH EXERCISES

Medicine Ball Crunch (Basic)

Targeted area: abdominus recti.

Hold the medicine ball with both hands close to the chest. Feet stay on the floor and eyes look up toward the ceiling. Raise the upper body, head and shoulder blades off the floor as a unit, pause and then slowly lower to the floor.

Suggested repetitions and weight: Repeat the crunches for 1 to 3 sets, 10 to 20 repetitions with a 3-5kg (6-12lb) medicine ball.

Overhead Pull-Up (Basic)

Targeted area: abdominus recti, anterior deltoid, tensor fascia lata, rectus femoris.

Lie flat on the floor with the arms extended overhead, knees bent and feet on the floor. Hold the ball firmly between your hands and keep the arms extended as you sit up. Slowly return to the floor, lowering the head, shoulders and the ball in unison.

Suggested repetitions and weight: Execute 1 to 3 sets of 10 to 15 repetitions with a 3-5kg (6-10lb) medicine ball.

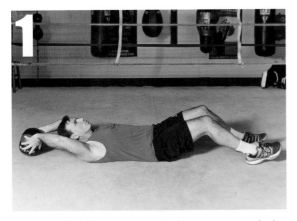

Overhead pull-up – start with the arms extended above your head.

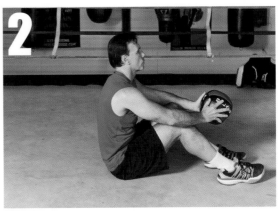

Overhead pull-up – finish with the ball by your legs.

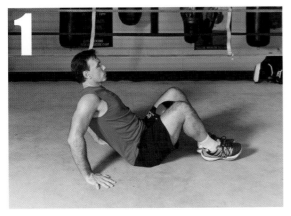

Seated bent-knee tuck – squeeze the ball firmly between your knees.

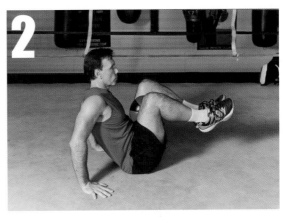

Seated bent-knee tuck – pull your knees towards your chest.

Seated Bent Knee Tuck (Basic)

Targeted area: abdominus recti, oblique abdominus externus, tensor fascia lata, rectus femoris.

Sit on the floor with the medicine ball placed between your knees. Keep the body in an upright position and lean back on your hands. Squeeze the ball firmly between your knees and then pull your knees and the ball in toward your chest. Next lower your knees and feet toward the floor. This is one repetition.

Suggested repetitions and weight: Execute 1 to 3 sets of 10 to 15 repetitions with a 3-5kg (6–10lb) medicine ball.

Side Pullover Sit-Up (Intermediate)

Targeted area: rectus abdominus, oblique abdominus externus, pec minor, anterior and medial deltoids.

Lie flat on the floor holding the medicine ball over the left shoulder. The ball is resting on the floor. As you sit up, pull the ball across the body and reach out to the right side. Always look at the ball and keep the movement smooth. Return to the start position and touch the ball on the floor by the shoulder. Keep looking at the ball. Execute the pullover on one side for the full number of repetitions and then duplicate the same number of repetitions on the other side.

Suggested repetitions and weight: Execute 1 to 2 sets of 10 to 15 repetitions with a 3–5kg (6–10lb) medicine ball.

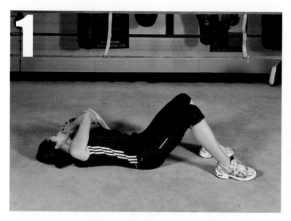

Side pullover – hold the ball close to your shoulder.

the medicine ball, arms, body and legs in a controlled, smooth manner back to the floor. Ensure that the legs are kept together and

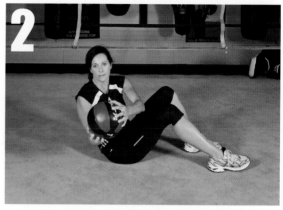

Side pullover – execute the pullover.

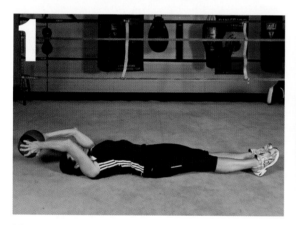

V-ups – start position.

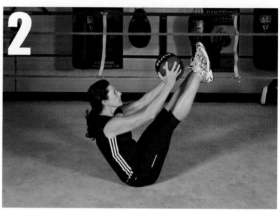

V-ups – lift the body and legs into a V-position.

V-Ups (Advanced)

Targeted area: abdominus recti, tensor fascia lata, rectus femoris, quadriceps.

This challenging move incorporates raising the upper body, arms and medicine ball simultaneously while lifting both legs. Start with the body flat on the floor, legs extended long and arms overhead. Hold the medicine ball with a firm grip. In one movement, lift the upper body and the legs into a V-position, reaching the ball to touch the feet. Pause and then lower

the arms stay straight and close to the head throughout the movement.

Option: Single Leg V-Up: An easier option is a single leg V-up. Leave one straight leg on the floor while you lift the other leg at the same time as you raise the body and arms. Reach and touch the ball to the elevated foot. The single leg V-up is easier as less stress is placed on the lower back muscles.

Suggested repetitions and weight: Execute 2 to 3 sets of 10 to 15 repetitions with a 3–4kg (6–8lb) medicine ball.

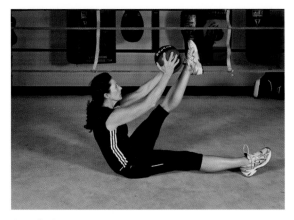

Single leg V-up – option.

Roll-Up and Knee Tuck (Advanced)

Targeted area: abdominus recti, tensor fascia lata, rectus femoris, quadriceps.

Lie flat on your back with your legs extended long. Hold the medicine ball between both hands above your head and slightly off the floor. Raise your arms and the ball at the same time as you raise your body and bring both knees in toward the chest. Reach the ball over the knees as if to hug them. Return slowly to the start position. Lower the body and arms at the same time as you extend the legs to a position just above the floor. Hold the legs extended a few centimetres off the floor until the next repetition.

Option: Single Leg Roll-Up and Knee Tuck: If this movement is too difficult, tuck one knee at a time and allow the opposite leg to rest on the floor. Alternate your legs with each repetition.

Suggested repetitions and weight: Execute 2 to 3 sets of 10 to 15 repetitions with a 3–4kg (6–8lb) medicine ball.

Medicine Ball Abdominal Press (Intermediate)

Targeted area: abdominus recti, oblique abdominus externus, tensor fascia lata, rectus femoris.

Sit on the floor holding the medicine ball at chest level. Start with the knees close to the chest and then slowly press both legs out, holding them just above the floor. Let the body move slightly backward as your legs are extended out. Pause and then pull the knees back toward the chest. Repeat.

Option: To make this exercise easier, do not hold onto the ball. Lean back and place your hands on the floor behind you with your fingertips facing forward and the elbows slightly bent.

Suggested repetitions and weight: Aim to complete 2 to 3 sets of 15 repetitions, holding a 3–5kg (6–10lb) medicine ball.

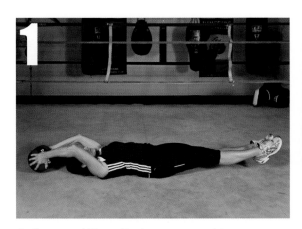

Roll-up and Knee Tuck – start position.

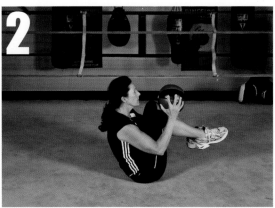

Roll-up and Knee Tuck – raise arms and legs in a smooth motion.

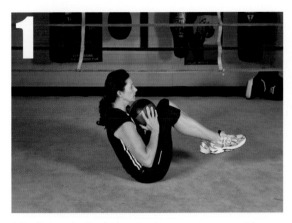

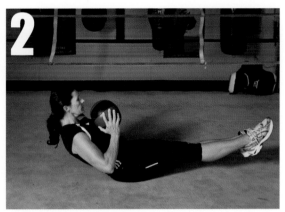

Medicine ball abdominal press – start with your knees in.

Press your legs long.

Medicine Ball Plank (Advanced)

Targeted area: rectus abdominus, oblique abdominus externus, serratus anterior.

Place both hands on the medicine ball and obtain the push-up position. Maintain a strong core by pulling the abs up toward the spine. The medicine ball plank is more difficult to perform than a regular plank because the medicine ball provides a very unstable base. More abdominal muscle fibres will be activated to maintain your balance when using the ball compared to supporting yourself on the floor with your elbows and forearms.

Suggested repetitions and weight: Try to hold for 30 seconds, increasing to 60 seconds. Repeat two to three times

Option: Plank without the medicine ball. Bend your elbows at 90 degrees with your body weight on your forearms. Keep your body flat, legs long and your shoulders directly above your elbows.

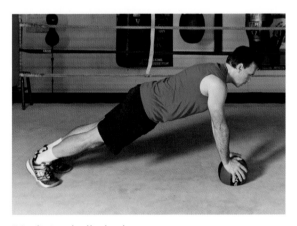

Medicine ball plank.

Medicine Ball Cycle (Intermediate)

Targeted area: abdominus externus, rectus abdominus, oblique abdominus, rectus femoris.

Sit on the floor holding the medicine ball tight to your chest. Move the legs in a cycling motion as you rotate your upper body; bring the left knee in toward the chest and rotate the body to the left, aiming to touch the right elbow on the left thigh; simultaneously extend the right leg just above the floor. Switch legs and bring the right knee toward the chest rotating your upper body to the right, touching the left elbow to the right thigh and extending the left leg above the floor. The movement of the ball from the left side to the right side and the right side to the left side (with the legs cycling) counts as one repetition. Ensure the movement is a slow, controlled and continuous motion.

Suggested repetitions and weight: Perform 2 to 3 sets of 20 to 30 repetitions, holding a 3–5kg (6–10lb) medicine ball.

back straight, shoulders relaxed and your head facing forward. Lower into a squat position, with your body weight centred through the feet and slightly onto your heels. Pause in the squat and then blast upward, pushing off the floor and extending the legs. When landing, roll through the balls of the feet and return to the squat position.

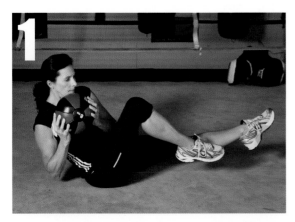

Medicine ball cycle – rotate the ball to the side.

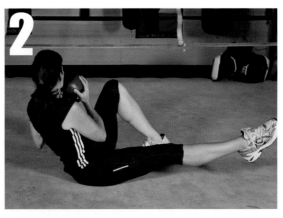

Move the legs in a cycling motion.

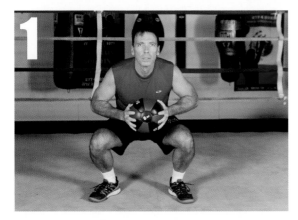

Power squat – lower into a squat position.

LOWER BODY EXERCISES

Power Squats (Advanced)

Targeted area: gluteus maximus, gluteus medius, quadriceps, soleus, gastroncnemius, plantaris.

Stand with the feet shoulder-width apart and the ball held in tight at chest level. Keep the

Blast upward.

Suggested repetitions and weight: Perform 1 to 2 sets, 10 to 15 repetitions, holding a 3–5kg (6–12lb) medicine ball.

180s (Advanced)

Targeted area: gluteus maximus, gluteus medius, quadriceps, soleus, gastroncnemius, plantaris.

This explosive move starts from a squat position with your feet positioned slightly wider than your shoulders. Hold the medicine ball at chest level, looking straight ahead with the shoulders relaxed and down, and placing your weight through the centre of your feet. Using the power of your legs, drive up into the air and turn 180 degrees, landing in a squat position facing in the opposite direction. Land softly and controlled, allowing the knees to absorb the impact. Alternate the direction of the turns, turning right then left.

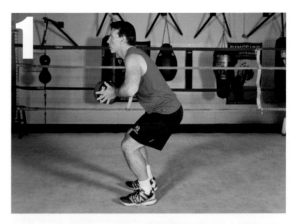

180s – start in a squat position.

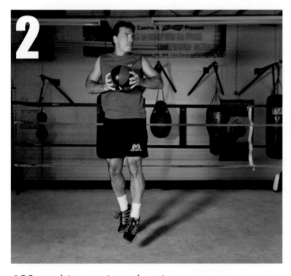

180s – drive up into the air.

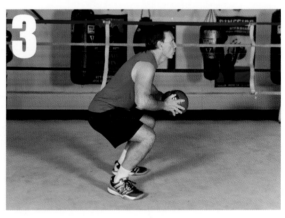

180s – land in a squat position.

Suggested repetitions and weight: Perform 2 to 3 sets, 12 to 15 repetitions or for 20-40 seconds, using a 3-4kg (6-8lb) medicine ball.

Forward Lunges (Intermediate)

Targeted area: gluteus maximus, quadriceps, biceps femoris.

Hold the medicine ball at chest level and feet side-by-side, shoulder width apart. Take a step forward with the left foot, planting the heel on

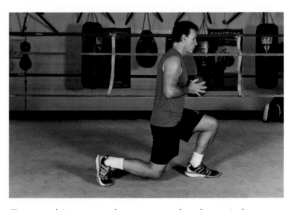

Forward Lunge – lower your body weight on the front leg.

the floor first. Lower your body weight onto the front leg ensuring the knee does not bend more than 90 degrees. Hold the core tight and perpendicular to your front thigh as the back knee bends toward the floor, acting as a stabilizer. Push off the front foot, firmly returning back to the start position. Repeat stepping forward with the other foot.

Suggested repetitions and weight: Perform 2 to 3 sets, 10 to 20 repetitions for each leg, using a 4–7kg (8–15lb) medicine ball.

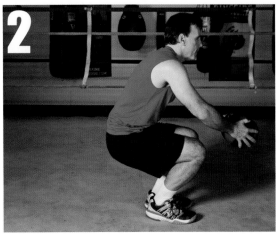

Roll up to your feet.

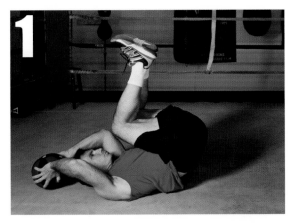

Rock and roll-up – roll backward and build momentum.

FULL BODY EXERCISES

Rock and Roll-up (Advanced)

Targeted area: gluteus maximus, quadriceps, biceps femoris, abdominus recti, anterior deltoid, tensor fascia lata, rectus femoris.

This challenging move works all the major muscle groups. Start lying on your back with your arms extended overhead holding a medicine ball. Tuck the knees in toward your chest, rolling backward and building momentum. Rock the body and swing the arms and ball forward. Roll up and finishing the move standing straight. Reverse the movement, lowering slowly into a squat, then onto your seat and returning onto your back. Keep your arms extended overhead with the ball.

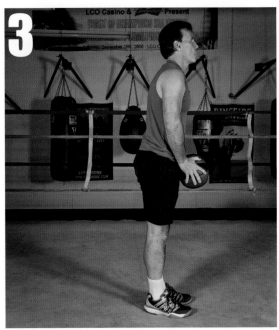

Rock and roll-up – finish standing straight.

Suggested repetitions and weight: Perform 2 to 3 sets, for 10 to 12 repetitions, holding a 3–4kg (6–8lb) medicine ball.

Medicine Ball Burpees (Advanced)

Targeted area: gluteus maximus, quadriceps, biceps femoris, abdominus recti, erector spinae, pectoralis major, serratus anterior, triceps.

The medicine ball stays on the floor. Rest both hands on the ball, lean forward and place your weight on the ball. From a squat position thrust your legs backward as far as possible, keeping the body long and strong, and hands steady on the ball. Jump in returning to the squat position and then jump into the air. Place your hands on the ball again ready to repeat the burpee.

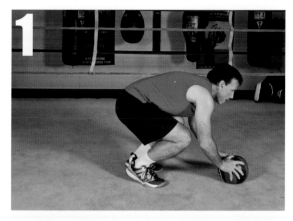

Medicine ball burpee – place your weight on the ball.

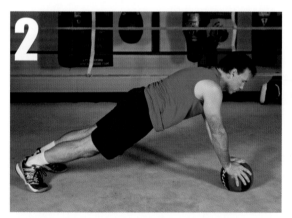

Medicine ball burpee – thrust your legs backwards.

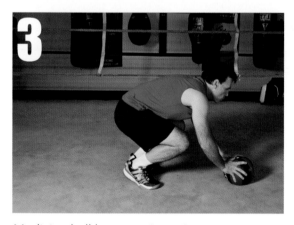

Medicine ball burpee – jump in.

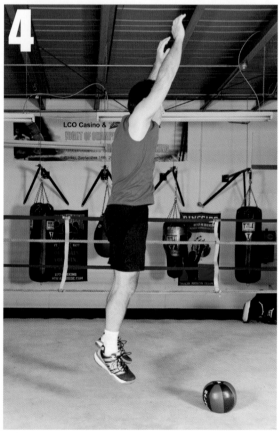

Medicine ball burpee – jump up.

Suggested repetitions and weight: Perform 2 to 3 sets, 12 to 15 repetitions. Select a medicine ball that is larger in size to give you a more stable bas

Woodchopper (Intermediate)

Targeted area: gluteus maximus, quadriceps, biceps femoris, abdominus recti, erector spinae, oblique abdominus exertnus, latissimus dorsi, deltoids, biceps brachii.

Standing with your feet slightly wider than shoulder width apart and your arms extended, hold the medicine ball overhead. Bend the body forward, mimicking a woodchopping motion, maintaining a secure grip on the ball. Allow the ball to fall toward the floor and between your legs and then quickly bring the ball back up to the start position. This is one repetition.

Suggested repetitions and weight: Perform 2 to 3 sets, 10 to 12 repetitions, holding a 3-4kg (6-8lb) medicine ball.

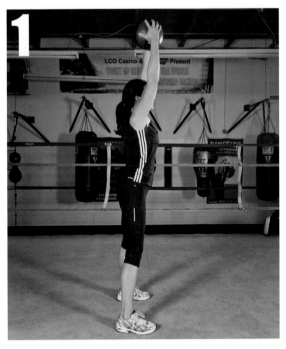

Woodchopper – hold the ball overhead.

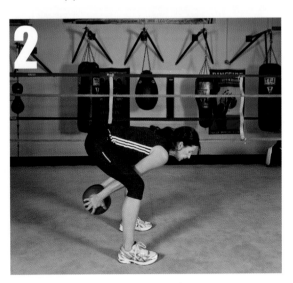

Swing the ball between your legs.

Mountain Climber (Intermediate)

Targeted area: gluteus maximus, quadriceps, biceps femoris , abdominus recti, erector spinae.

Place the medicine ball on the floor, with your hands firmly gripping the ball. Lower your body and perform a running leg motion, moving your feet back and forth.

Suggested repetitions and weight: Perform 2 to 3 sets, 12 to 15 repetitions or for 20–40 seconds. Select a medicine ball that is larger in size to give you a more stable base.

Choose the exercises you prefer to perform for each area of the body and execute the exercises smoothly and with control. The medicine ball exercises described will increase your muscular strength and endurance, and are part of the complete Fitness Boxing workout in Chapter 10.

Key Points: Medicine Ball

- Ensure you have a secure grip on the ball.
- Reduce the weight of the ball if you feel any pain in the joint areas.
- Use a larger sized medicine ball when balancing on the ball.
- Exhale on exertion or when pressing or pushing the medicine ball away from the body.
- Inhale when returning the medicine ball back to the start position.

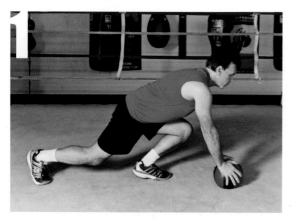
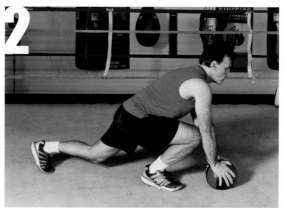

Mountain Climber – have a firm grip on the ball.

Alternate your legs in a running motion.

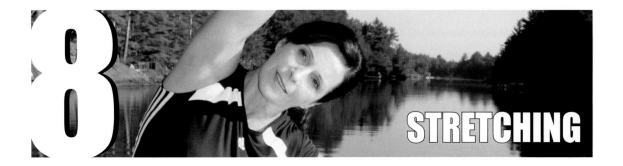

With the normal ageing process flexibility decreases, muscles shorten in length, and good posture and balance are compromised. Limb and joint movement is reduced and full range of motion is often restricted. Muscles and joints also lose their extensibility, and you become more predisposed to muscle tears, injuries and muscle soreness. A regular stretching programme is essential to maintain the best possible conditioned and flexible musculature and the optimal range of motion at your joints. Including a stretching session in all your workouts gives you a sound and effective training programme.

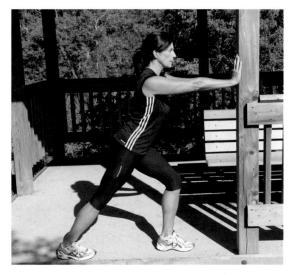

Flexible muscles enhance athletic performance.

IMPORTANCE OF STRETCHING

Improving Athletic Performance
Good flexibility is essential for everyday living, and with respect to sports and training, it is especially valuable in enhancing athletic performance. Optimal muscle length and joint mobility provide better coordination and muscle control, and allow for proper execution of movements. When the overall length of a relaxed muscle is increased, the power and the elasticity in the muscle are intensified. To perform with efficiency and effectiveness the strength and the extensibility of a muscle must be proportionate.

Reduction of Injuries
Stretching increases blood flow to the muscles and helps improve circulation. The more conditioned and subtle your muscles and tendons are, the better they can manage intense physical demands. Flexible joints and limbs can per

form a movement travelling a greater distance before an injury will occur. A strong muscle that is pliable and limber can withstand any additional stress resulting from intense training. A strong muscle that is rigid and inflexible will tear, resulting in soreness and discomfort.

Reduction of Muscle Soreness
Increased blood flow to the muscle tissues supplies essential nutrients to working muscles and helps to reduce muscle soreness. The lactic acid that builds up in the muscle tissue when you are working out will often cause soreness and fatigue in your muscles. By stretching these muscles, the blood circulation to that area is increased and helps to flush out the lactic acid build-up. By lowering the occurrence of muscle soreness, you are more likely to stick with your workout schedule.

STRETCHING BASICS

Take Time to Stretch

Focus on the key areas that you are training and include more stretches for these areas. Be aware of the muscles that are tight and spend additional time stretching them. Often people will not stretch a muscle or joint area until they actually feel stiff or sore. Aim to find the balance between the strength of a muscle and the extensibility of that same muscle. Due to sport-specific demands, poor postural habits or previous injuries muscular imbalance may be evident. Take the time to stretch the muscles that have become too tight or inflexible. Stretch both sides of your body making sure that the range of motion and extensibility are as equal as possible on each side.

Even though it is most beneficial to perform stretching exercises at the end of your workout, you may be tired and less enthusiastic to do so and may forgo your stretching. Over a period of time this often leads to the muscles becoming less pliable and a reduced range of motion at your joint areas. Always make time to stretch with every workout and become aware of your body and musculature by stretching in relaxed surroundings.

Pre-Activity Stretch

The purpose of a pre-activity stretch is to warm up the muscles and joint areas and not necessarily to increase the length of the muscle. Before performing stretches always warm up your muscles and joint areas by increasing your heart rate. This can be accomplished by walking around, performing large arm circles and leg lifts, or imitating the training you will be doing later, for about 5 minutes. Then stretch your muscles to reduce any tightness and hold the stretches for 5–15 seconds.

Post-Activity Stretch

The purpose of a post-activity stretch is to lengthen the muscles you have been training. Hold a post-activity stretch for 30–60 seconds, moving into the stretch until a mild tension is felt in the muscle, pause and then try to reach slightly further into the stretch. Always move gently and slowly into the stretch. If it feels painful, then you have moved into the stretch too far or too fast. Release the stretch and hold at the point where there is not any pain.

Focus on the muscle you are trying to lengthen and do not place any stress on the associated joints. Never bounce or force a stretch, as this can cause small tears in the muscle fibres, resulting in pain and scar tissue. Always breathe during your stretch and never hold your breath. Breathe in as you prepare for the stretch and breathe out as you move into your stretch.

Perform stretches for all of your muscle groups, spending additional time stretching the muscles you have trained hard and any muscles that feel tight.

UPPER BODY STRETCHES

Neck Stretch

Targeted area: levator scapula, upper trapezius.

Either sitting or standing, bend your head to the right side and slightly forward. Place the left hand lightly on the side of your head, and gently pull downward. Hold the stretch for 30 seconds. Release and perform the stretch tilting your head to the left side.

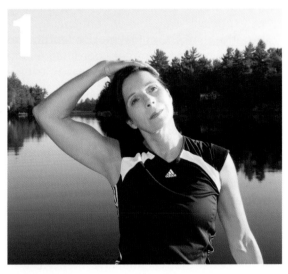

Neck stretch – tilt your head to one side.

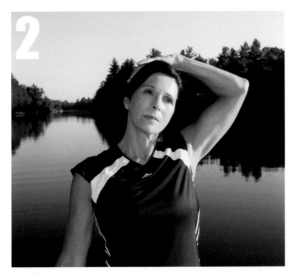

Next bend the right arm at the elbow, inhale and then exhale pressing the arm across your chest toward the left shoulder. Allow the shoulder to roll forward slightly. This stretches out the rear deltoid muscle of the shoulder. Hold the stretch for 30 seconds. Release. Perform both stretches with each arm.

Neck stretch – gently stretch on opposite side.

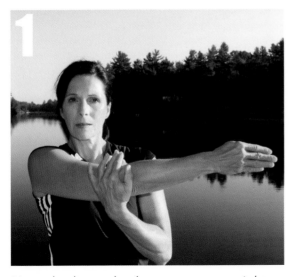

Upper back stretch – keep your arm straight.

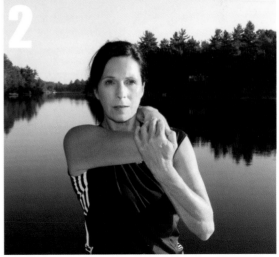

Shoulder stretch – bent at the elbow and press back.

Upper Back and Shoulder Stretch

Targeted area: trapezius, rhomboid, teres minor, teres major, infraspinatus, posterior deltoid.

To stretch the upper back, extend the right arm and bring it in front of your body. Keep the shoulders square and relaxed, and hold onto the elbow area with your left hand. Take a breath and as you exhale gently press the arm toward your body. Hold the stretch for 30-seconds. Release.

Pull Back Lat Stretch

Targeted area: latissimus dorsi, posterior deltoid, infraspinatus.

Standing, grasp a secure object that is fixed to the floor or ground with both hands at approximately waist level. Breathe in, and then exhale as you sit back allowing the arms to fully extend, stretching through the latissimus dorsi and posterior deltoid. Try shifting your weight slightly to one side for a further stretch in the back region. Hold the stretch for 30 seconds breathing naturally.

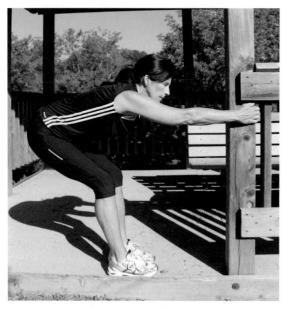

Pull back lat stretch – exhale as you sit back.

Chest and Shoulder Stretch

Targeted area: pectoralis major, pectoralis minor, anterior deltoid.

To stretch the chest and shoulder muscles, stand with your head facing straight forward and your neck and shoulders relaxed. Extend your arms behind your back and hold your hands together by interlacing the fingers. Inhale, pull the shoulder blades toward each other and lift the arms up slightly. Now exhale and lower the arms down slowly. Hold the stretch for 30 seconds.

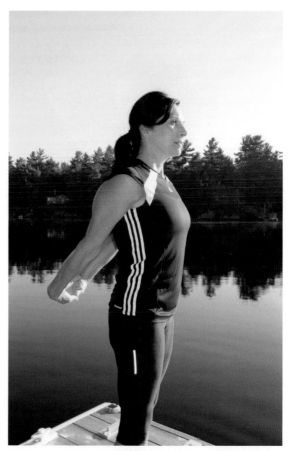

Chest and shoulder stretch – keep your neck and shoulders relaxed.

Overhead Triceps Stretch

Targeted area: triceps, deltoid, rotator cuff.

The triceps, deltoids and rotator cuff are all stretched with this exercise. Both arms start in the overhead position. Look forward with the head in a frontal neutral position. Bend the right arm back with the elbow pointing toward the ceiling. Try to place the palm of the right hand or your fingers near the centre of your back, between the shoulder blades. Place your left hand on the elbow, breathe in and then as you breathe out, press down on the elbow slightly moving the hand down the back. Hold the stretch for 30 seconds. Release the stretch. Repeat with the left arm.

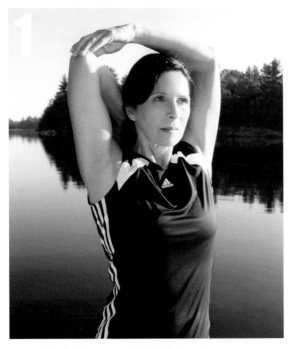

Overhead triceps stretch – front view.

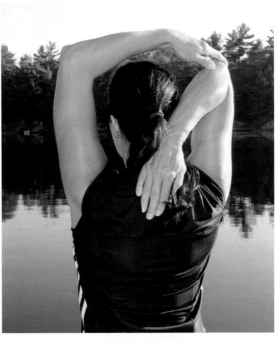

Overhead triceps stretch – back view.

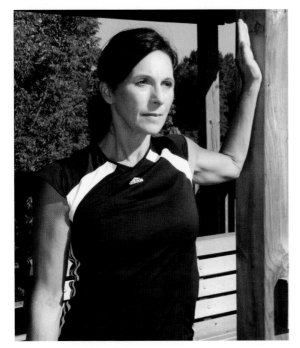

Chest and biceps stretch – allow your muscles to relax completely.

Chest and Biceps Stretch

Targeted area: pectoralis major, pectoralis minor, biceps, rotator cuff, deltoids.

Standing by a wall, place your bent left arm at shoulder height against the wall. Breathe in, and then exhale slowly as you turn your body away from the wall. To target the upper chest muscles place the arm further down on the wall, and to target the lower chest muscle place your arm in a position that is slightly higher on the wall. Hold the stretch for 30-60 seconds. Release the stretch. Repeat with the right arm.

Kneeling Forearm Stretch

Targeted area: brachioradialis, palmaris longus, flexor carpi radialis.

Kneeling with your arms directly positioned under your shoulders, press the palms of your hands into the ground with the fingers spread apart. Lift the right hand and rotate it outward, keeping the fingers spread. Press your palm into the ground and circle your arm at the shoulder joint slowly in one direction for about 10 seconds, and then change direction. Breathe normally. Release the stretch and repeat with the left arm.

Alternate: This stretch may be executed while you are standing or sitting by holding onto the palm of the right hand with the left and lightly pressing backward. Hold the stretch for 30 seconds. Release the stretch. Repeat with the left arm.

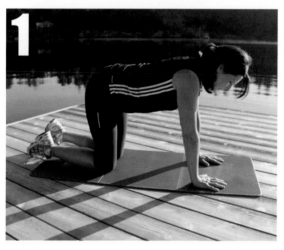

Kneeling forearm stretch – arms directly under your shoulders.

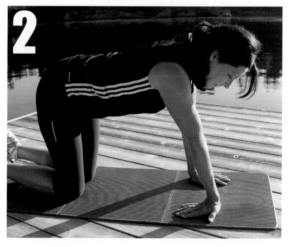

Kneeling forearm stretch – press the palms of your hands into the ground.

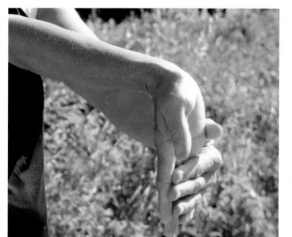

Alternate – standing forearm stretch.

Core Side Stretch

Targeted area: rectus abdominus, obliques, latissimus dorsi.

Stand with the feet shoulder width apart, hipbones parallel to the ground, abdominal muscles held tight and your knees slightly bent. Inhale, and then stretch your right arm overhead, exhaling as you reach your arm in a semicircle and bending your body to the left side. Feel the stretch from your fingertips through to your hipbone. Breathe normally, holding the side stretch for 30-60 seconds. Take a breath in and then exhale, reaching up and returning to the start position. Repeat on the other side.

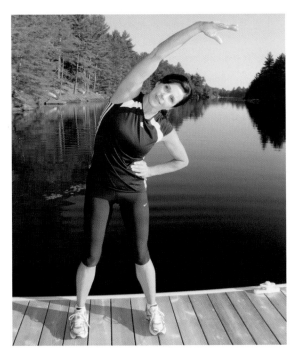

Core side stretch – gently stretch to the side.

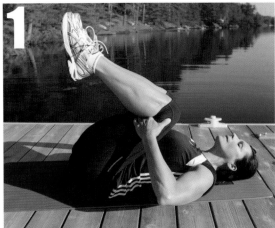

Lower back stretch – pull both knees to your chest.

LOWER BODY STRETCHES

Lower Back Stretch

Targeted area: erector spinae, gluteals.

To stretch your lower back and gluteal area, lie on your back with your knees bent and both feet on the ground. Breathe in, and then exhale as you pull both of your knees in toward your chest, clasping behind your knees. Hold the stretch for 30 seconds. Slowly release the legs and place both feet back on the floor.

You can vary the stretch by starting with both knees in by your chest, inhale and then as you exhale extend the left leg long on the ground. Hold the stretch for 30 seconds. Bring both legs back to the chest and repeat with the right leg.

To reduce the stress on your lower back, just pull one knee in toward the chest with your other foot on the floor.

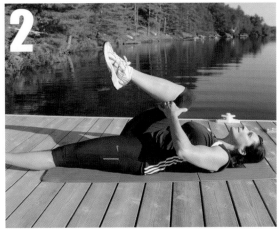

Lower back stretch – keep one knee by the chest as you extend your other leg.

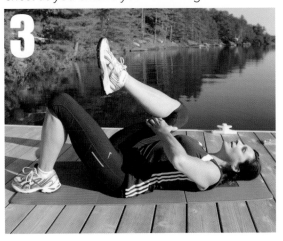

Lower back stretch – keep one foot on the floor.

Supine Piriformis Stretch

Targeted area: piriformis, gluteals, fascia lata.

This stretch helps prevent lower back tightening and tension. Start by lying on your back with your knees bent and the left foot on the ground. Place the ankle of the right leg on the left bent knee. Lift both legs off the ground holding behind the thigh of the lower leg. Inhale and as you exhale, pull your legs in toward the chest. Breathe normally, holding the stretch for 30 seconds. Release and repeat on the other side.

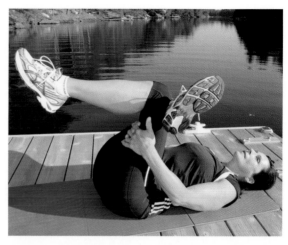

Supine piriformis stretch – pull the knees toward the chest.

Kneeling Hip Flexor Stretch

Targeted area: hip flexors, quadriceps, groin.

To stretch a tight hip flexor muscle, place the left knee on the ground and the right foot in front on the ground, ensuring that the front foot is positioned directly under the knee and the hip is bent at 90 degrees. Look forward with the head in a frontal neutral position and place both hands on your right thigh, keeping your back straight. Inhale and as you breathe out lightly press your hips forward. Hold the stretch for 30 seconds. Release and repeat on the other side.

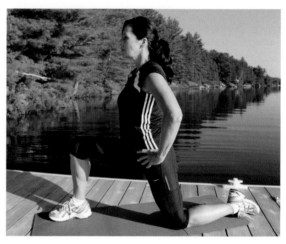

Kneeling hip flexor stretch – lightly press your hip forward.

Standing Quadriceps Stretch

Targeted area: quadriceps, rectus femoris.

To stretch the front of your thighs, stand with your back and torso straight and thighs together. Lift your left foot backward and upward, keeping the knees close together. Take a breath in and hold onto your left ankle with your left hand. Exhale pulling the heel up and toward your buttock. Hold this position for 30 seconds. Gently release and repeat on the other side.

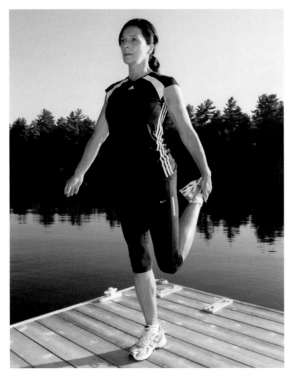

Standing quadriceps stretch – lift one foot backward.

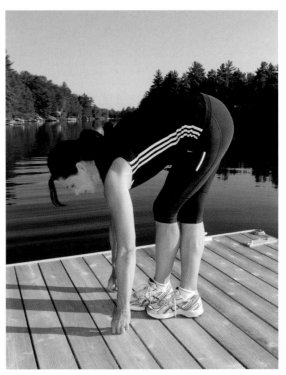

ITB stretch – exhale as you reach forward.

ITB Stretch

Targeted area: iliotibial band, tensor fascia lata.

The iliotibial band is a thick band of connective tissue runs along the outer thigh from the hip area to the knee. When it is not flexible and pliable, the knee joint may be pulled out of alignment and cause inflammation in your hip area. Stand and cross your left foot over your right foot, keeping the knees soft or unlocked. Inhale, bending at the waist and exhale as you reach toward the floor. To increase the stretch, centre your weight through the rear leg. Hold this position for 30 seconds. Gently release and switch legs.

Lying Hamstring Stretch

Targeted area: hamstrings, erector spinae, gluteals.

Start the hamstring stretch by lying on your back with both knees bent. Lift your right leg and hold behind the thigh with both of your hands. Inhale and then exhale while you straighten the leg. Slowly pull the leg toward your body until a slight tension is felt in the hamstring muscle. Hold this position for 30 seconds. Gently release and switch legs. For a deeper stretch keep both legs extended long on the ground and lift the right leg up and toward your body. Hold for 30 seconds and repeat with the other leg.

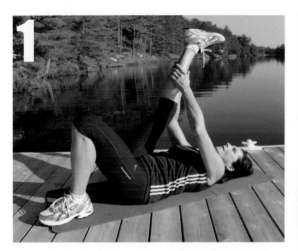

Lying hamstring stretch – slowly pull your leg toward your body.

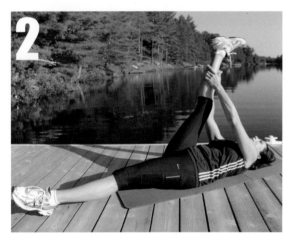

Lying hamstring stretch – for deeper stretch keep your legs extended.

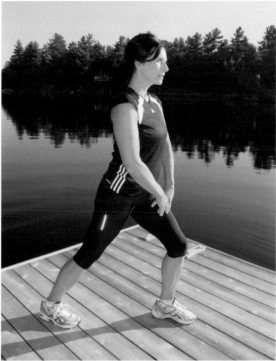

Standing calf/Achilles stretch – keep your heel on the ground.

Standing Calf/Achilles Stretch

Targeted area: gastrocnemius, Achilles tendon.

Stand with the right leg forward and the left leg back. Inhale and as you bend the right leg forward, exhale, keeping your left leg straight and the heel on the ground. The stretch will be felt in the centre of the left calf muscle. To stretch the lower area of the calf, bend your left knee slightly and shift your body weight back over the heel. This will stretch through the lower part of the gastrocnemius muscle and the Achilles tendon area of the left leg. Hold each position

Kneeling Soleus/Achilles Stretch

Targeted area: soleus, Achilles tendon.

Start with the left knee on the ground and the right foot placed on the ground beside your left knee. Position your hands slightly in front of the knee on the ground to assist with balancing. Try to position your heel as close to the knee as possible. Take a breath in, and as you exhale press your right heel to the ground and shift your body weight forward slightly onto your hands. Hold this position for 30 seconds. Gently release and switch legs.

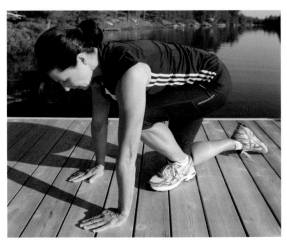

Kneeling soleus/Achilles stretch – position your heel close to your knee.

STRETCHING ROUTINES

Stretching is an important part of a complete fitness programme. It is advisable to cool down and stretch after every workout. Below are two options: an 8-minute stretch routine and a more extensive 15-minute stretch routine. Take your time to perform these exercises in the order laid out. Include the 15-minute routine in your training schedule, two to three times per week.

8-Minute Routine (9 Stretches)

1. Upper Back and Shoulder Stretch
2. Pull Back Lat Stretch
3. Chest and Biceps Stretch
4. Forearm Stretch
5. Piriformis Stretch
6. Kneeling Hip Flexor Stretch
7. Standing Quadriceps Stretch
8. Hamstring Stretch
9. Standing Calf/Achilles Stretch

15-Minute Routine (16 Stretches)

1. Neck Stretch
2. Upper Back and Shoulder Stretch
3. Pull Back Lat Stretch
4. Chest and Shoulder Stretch
5. Triceps Stretch
6. Chest and Biceps Stretch
7. Forearm Stretch
8. Core Side Stretch
9. Lower Back Stretch
10. Piriformis Stretch
11. Kneeling Hip Flexor Stretch
12. Standing Quadriceps Stretch
13. ITB Stretch
14. Hamstring Stretch
15. Standing Calf/Achilles Stretch
16. Soleus/Achilles Stretch

Key Points: Stretching

- Never bounce when you are stretching. Muscles, tendons and ligaments can be stressed and result in injury.
- A static stretch, when a muscle is lengthened just beyond its natural length and held for more than 30 seconds, is the safest and most effective method of stretching.
- Do not force a muscle to over stretch. Once a tension is felt in the muscle, ease off and hold the length at the point where there is not any discomfort.

Improvements in your flexibility, muscle length and joint mobility will be noticeable if you stretch on a regular basis. Remember, stretching should not feel painful. If there is pain associated with your stretches ensure you are executing the movements correctly. If you have any joint problems or issues with your back or neck consult with your doctor before performing the exercises.

FUEL YOUR WORKOUT

A boxer's training routine is strenuous and often long, with a morning session of roadwork followed by an afternoon session of sparring and bag work. One way a competitive boxer can gain an advantage over an opponent is by adhering to a good diet, full of high-quality nutrition and available fuel. Whatever sports or activities you are involved in, you need to fuel your workouts to get the maximum results.

A healthy diet not only provides a strong foundation to build a healthy lifestyle, it also delivers the energy required for an optimal workout. Our bodies continually undergo a building and renewal cycle on a daily basis and we need to eat good carbohydrates, proteins and fats each day to provide nutrition for muscle repair, growth and energy. A smart and healthy diet reduces body fat (not just a reduction in water), helps to improve cardiovascular health, reduces the risk of heart disease, hypertension and cancer, and gives energy to perform normal daily activities. It provides the fuel for you to train at an optimal workout level, giving you the best possible results. Your performance and power output are dependent on your nutritional habits.

To workout at your optimum and to improve your fitness level you need to include carbohydrates, proteins and essential fats in your diet every day. Carbohydrates are required for energy, proteins are needed to repair and develop musculature, and the essential fats are necessary to assist in the absorption of specific vitamins and minerals and to regulate hormonal activity.

THE THREE BASIC FUELS

Carbohydrates

Carbohydrates are needed to provide the precious energy that enables you to continue and finish a workout. Foods consisting of complex carbohydrates have higher fibre contents and break down slower in your system. This provides energy at a slower rate over a longer period of time while you are training.

Simple carbohydrates, like white sugar, processed grains, commercial cereals, bananas and raisins break down quickly and will give a quick burst of energy, but then quickly leave you feeling depleted. When carbohydrates are converted into blood sugar or blood glucose, the hormone insulin transports the blood glucose to the liver and muscle tissue and it is stored as glycogen. This stored glycogen provides energy for about two hours and then it is converted into fat and stored as fat.

Carbohydrates should make up 40 per cent of your daily food intake. Choose complex carbohydrates like apples, grapes, grapefruit, beans, legumes, nuts, seeds and whole grain cereal, pasta and bread to eat.

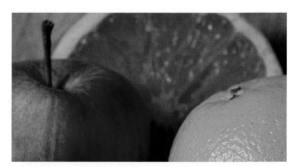

Eat to fuel your workouts.

Proteins

High effort training means you will be breaking down muscle fibres and you will experience muscle soreness. Protein is necessary in your diet as it assists in repairing the torn muscle fibres, developing new muscle fibre growth, producing hormones, antibodies and vital enzymes, and assisting in metabolizing fats. When an adequate amount of protein is ingested you will reduce the amount of muscle soreness experienced after your workout and physiological benefits will be noted. It is on your rest days that the majority of the repairing and new growth of your muscle fibres occurs.

Good protein sources are chicken breast, turkey breast, egg whites, tuna, tofu and supplementary protein shakes. Proteins should make up 30 per cent of your daily food intake.

Fats

Specific dietary fats need to be included in your diet. The essential unsaturated fats are known as fatty acids. Omega-3 and omega-6 fatty acids help to regulate a number of your bodily functions like lowering the risk of heart attacks, strokes and diabetes. Good fat sources are salmon, tuna, olive oil and flaxseed oil. Saturated fats, such as fried foods and hydrogenated oils should only be eaten in moderation.

It is also important to have fatty tissue on and in the body to stay alive. Fat protects the vital organs, stores energy, insulates the body and contributes with the transportation and absorption of some vitamins. Dietary fats should make up 30 per cent of your daily food intake.

MICRO-NUTRIENTS

While the following three nutrients do not give us the basic energy to perform they are necessary in our daily diets.

Vitamins

Vitamins cannot be made within the body, so eating a diet including a variety of food types helps to ensure you are getting the sufficient amount and type of vitamins to stay healthy. Thirteen vitamins are necessary for normal growth, regulating essential bodily functions and building and maintaining bones, teeth, skin and blood. A deficiency in vitamins can damage your health. Conversely an excess of certain vitamins can also be harmful.

Fat-soluble vitamins, like A, D, E and K are stored in our bodies within the liver and fatty tissue and can be toxic if taken in high doses. Water-soluble vitamins, like C, B-vitamins and H, are not stored in the body and need to be replenished daily. Vitamin supplements are often recommended in certain medically defined situations such as: a proven vitamin deficiency, a risk of a deficiency or a reduced capacity to absorb a vitamin. However eating a well-balanced diet provides the most beneficial method of getting the vitamin you need.

Minerals

Minerals are required for our bodies to work properly, to assist with growth and development, and are important for building strong bones and teeth, and having healthy blood and hair as well as nerve and muscle function. All minerals are essential for your health and are obtained by eating a variety of nutritious foods and drinking healthy fluids.

Minerals such as sodium, potassium, calcium and magnesium are known as macro-minerals and are needed on a daily basis and in a larger amount. These specific minerals set up the basis for electrical impulses that travel along your nerves and muscles, and without them athletic performance is compromised. The minerals that are required in smaller amounts and less often are known as micro-minerals or trace elements and include zinc, copper, iron, iodine, sulphur and chloride.

Salt

Salt (sodium chloride) is often the electrolyte that is lost during training and needs to be replenished. A salty snack (crisps, pretzel, sports drink) will assist in your recovery.

Water

In order to survive and keep your body functioning well, it is essential that you include water in your diet. Water is packed with minerals and electrolytes and it keeps you hydrated by replacing what is lost when you sweat and urinate. The body is made up of 50-70 per cent water, while the brain is 80 per cent water.

Water helps you digest food, dissolves nutrients so they can be absorbed into your blood stream, and carries waste products out of your body. Water helps to regulate your body temperature by perspiring. It acts a lubricant for your joints, assists with the digestion of food, production of energy, building of new tissue, and sending electrical communication between the cells enabling your muscles to respond and produce a movement.

The majority of the water in your body is intercellular. The correct fluid balance between the intercellular fluid and the extracellular fluid (other body liquids like blood plasma, urine, the fluid between the cells, and lymph) must be in balance. If there is too little water in the cell, the cell will shrivel and die. Too much water will cause the cell to burst. You can live without food for two to four weeks but you can only live without water a matter of days. Always stay hydrated and drink before, during and after your training. Do not wait until you feel thirsty, as the dehydration process has already started.

CALORIES

Basic energy requirements are referred to as calories. The term 'calorie' is used to indicate the energy units that are ingested and also used or burned off for basic survival and activity.

It is important to know how many calories you are ingesting versus the number of calories you are burning off. The basal metabolic rate (BMR) is the amount of energy expended by humans while they are at rest. This energy (or the calories burned) sustains the functioning of your vital organs, such as the heart, lungs, kidneys, liver and intestines. Calories are also expended when performing physical activities. The more intense an activity, the more calories are burned.

Caloric Values

The caloric content of the three basic fuels, per gram:

Protein	4 calories
Carbohydrates	4 calories
Fat	9 calories

To be in a caloric balance, you should eat approximately the same number of calories as the body is using. In this case your body weight will remain stable. If you are in caloric excess, you are consuming more calories than your body is using and these extra calories will be stored as fat and show as a weight gain. If you are in a caloric deficit, you are consuming fewer calories than your body requires to remain at a stable weight, and you will show a weight loss.

The amount of calories required varies based on your age, sex and activity level. As you get older or if you live a sedentary lifestyle the recommended caloric intake decreases. The more physically active you are, the more calories you need to consume. The following chart is categorized into age groups and shows the acceptable number of calories that can be consumed per day for both men and women when performing normal daily activities. If you are more active, an extra 200 to 400 calories can be consumed.

Recommended Calories per Day

(for normal daily activity)

Men

14–18 years	2200 calories
19–30 years	2400
31–50 years	2200
51+	2000

Women

14–18 years	1800 calories
19–30 years	2000
31–50 years	1800
51 +	1600

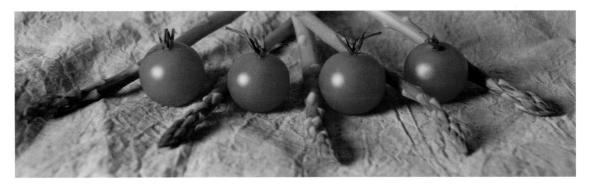

Choose your calories carefully.

Every person's body is unique and made up of varying proportions of fat, muscle and bone. Women generally have a smaller bone structure and a lower body mass than men and therefore require fewer calories for energy.

Increased physical activity levels and intense training requires a higher caloric intake to maintain a desired weight or girth measurement. It should also be noted that it takes more calories to sustain muscle tissue than fatty tissue. Someone with a greater muscle mass will be burning more calories performing a similar activity. This is one reason men can generally eat more calories than women and not gain weight. Due to the male hormonal influence, men have a greater muscle mass. By weight training, increases in muscle mass can be attained.

Counting calories sometimes assists you in understanding how much you are consuming. Keep a food diary and record the types of foods and beverages you are eating and drinking. The associated calories will give you a base as to whether you are consuming the correct number of calories to maintain your desired weight. There are a number of online calorie counters to help you keep track of your caloric intake.

The recommended weight loss per week is about 0.5–1kg (1–2lb). One kilogram has approximately 7700 calories. By reducing your caloric intake by 500–1000 calories per day, or by increasing your physical activity level and burning off 500–1000 calories per day you could lose about 0.5–1kg in a week.

VEGAN AND VEGETARIAN DIET CONCERNS

As a vegan you must be diligent about plant-based protein intake because of the elimination of the animal based proteins. It is important to include a good source of plant-based proteins and an adequate amount (60–90 grams per day) in your diet for the development of new muscle growth and muscle tissue repair.

The main issue facing those not including meat or dairy products is the non-existence of vitamin B12 in your diet, because it is only found in animal-based foods. B12 affects red blood cell production and it is the red blood cells that carry the necessary oxygen for endurance workouts. Many cereals and soymilk are fortified with B12 and provide this essential vitamin. A supplement is an option to consider.

Also plant-based iron is more difficult to absorb into your tissues than animal-based protein, but with the addition of vitamin C it is more easily absorbed. Eating oranges or other citrus fruit with iron-fortified foods, such as whole grain cereals, beans, tempeh, nuts and soy should provide you with sufficient amounts of iron.

A vegan/vegetarian's diet naturally includes sufficient carbohydrates and fats to fuel for training, and with the inclusion of good plant-based proteins a well balanced diet is realistic. As always, if you have any concerns about your nutritional status, it is best to consult with your doctor or a registered sports nutritionist.

Vegan/Vegetarian Limits

Vegans eliminate all animal products from their diet, including dairy, eggs and honey. Vegetarians eliminate meat, fish, poultry and products that contain gelatine or other meat-based products. Lacto-vegetarians consume dairy, but no eggs. Ovo-vegetarians eat eggs but not dairy products, and lacto-ovo vegetarians eat both eggs and dairy products.

WHEN TO EAT

Calories provide energy. Try to eat 30 per cent of your total calories between the time you get up and 10am, then 40 per cent during the middle of the day (10am to 3pm), and 30 per cent in the early evening (3pm to 8pm).

It is important to know how many calories you are ingesting versus the amount of fat-burning and muscle-building exercises you are performing. When athletes eat the correct number of calories from a variety of food groups, then vitamin/mineral supplements are not required. If you limit your caloric intake for a sport that requires a specific weight, like boxing, or eliminate a food group because of an intolerance like lactose, or a principle or belief like being a vegan, you may not eat a sufficient number of nutritious calories and may require supplements.

Eating Before Your Workout

Try to eat healthy carbohydrates 2 to 3 hours before your workout, usually about 300 to 500 calories. You will require this food for energy to get you through the workout. Eat food that agrees with your digestive system.

Fuel Your Performance

If you are exercising for less than an hour there is no need to eat during the workout. You will just want to ensure that you stay hydrated by drinking small sips of water often. If you were unable to eat before a workout, you may choose dried fruits, sport gels or sport drinks with protein as fuel during your performance. When training over an extended period of time, plan to eat 50–100 calories of carbohydrates about every half hour to supply you with sufficient fuel for a good performance.

Eating After Your Workout

Ideally, try to eat some recovery carbohydrates and proteins within 30 to 60 minutes after training. The carbohydrates will replace the used up muscle glycogen and the protein will repair the damaged muscle fibres. This is especially important for athletes who are training or competing again within six hours. Absorption of nutrients occurs up to 24 hours after a workout, although at a slower rate, and if you have a full day to recover before your next workout you do not have to be pre-occupied with refuelling immediately.

There are sport drinks and gels that offer a good carbohydrate/protein ratio of 4:1. An easy choice is chocolate milk, which contains both carbohydrates and protein. Vegans could choose a soy or almond milk option. Also, you can combine a carbohydrate like whole wheat bread (2 slices), with a protein like turkey (2oz) for a satisfactory refuelling, approximately 250–400 calories.

Key Points: Smart Choices

- Start the day by eating a healthy breakfast.
- Eat a nutritious midday meal.
- Snack on healthy food choices.
- Eat a smaller evening meal.
- Eat carbohydrates 2 to 3 hours before your training.
- After your workout, eat carbohydrates with some protein.
- Include some essential fatty acids in your daily diet.
- Stay hydrated drinking 8 to 10 glasses of water per day.

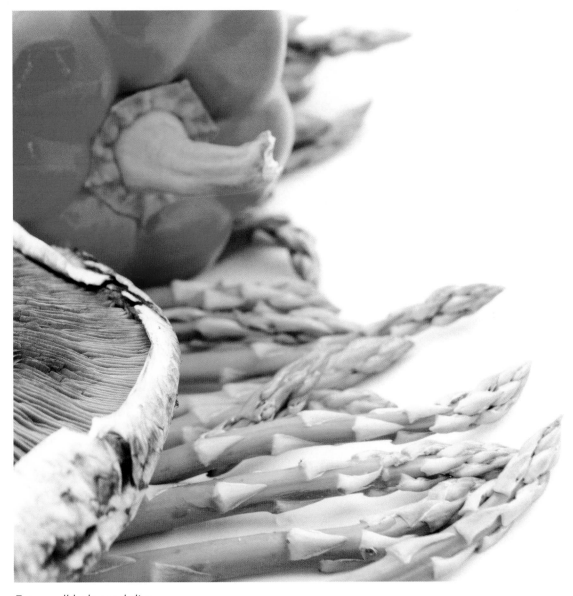

Eat a well balanced diet.

A Well-Balanced Diet

Without a well-balanced diet, your body is unable to meet the demands of a training regimen. Carbohydrates are needed for energy, protein for muscle growth and repair, and fats for providing essential nutrients and protection from diseases. If you follow a good diet your workout performance will improve, muscle soreness will be reduced, and you will become stronger, leaner and more physically fit.

Before going on a diet, consult with your doctor or a nutritional specialist. Be wary of fad diets, as often they do not provide the necessary nutrients and energy.

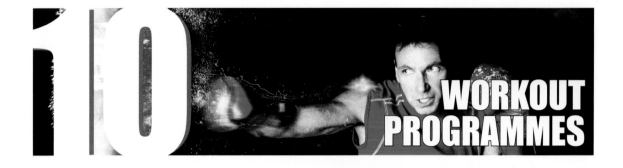

WORKOUT PROGRAMMES

This chapter brings together all the elements of boxing training and presents various training options. Three different levels are described for you to choose the appropriate workout depending on your current fitness level, past experience and training objectives. The first level is the basic workout. This workout is most beneficial for the novice fitness boxer and it is a workout that can easily compliment your existing training programme. The second level, the contender workout, adds more intensity to your training and requires a greater commitment to train like a boxer. Additional training elements are added to this workout and the skill level is increased. The third level, the champ's workout, is a serious commitment which requires dedication. The complexity of the drills and the intensity of the training are pushed to the maximum and you will require passion and dedication.

Easy to follow 12-week training programmes are described for the contender workout and the champ's workout, giving you specific training challenges selected from the multitude of exercises and drills described in the previous chapters. You will notice crossover benefits in other activities and improvements to your overall fitness level.

Use the Perceived Exertion Chart (Chapter 1) to ensure you are training at the desired level.

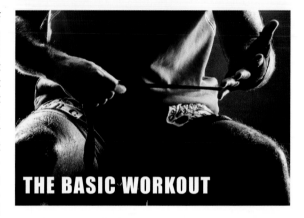

THE BASIC WORKOUT

(3-Day/Week Programme)

The basic workout is a great introduction to fitness boxing. It is designed so you can integrate fitness boxing it into your current fitness schedule. Perform the basic workout 3 days per week, every other day. This workout includes heavy bag, jumping rope, shadow boxing, focus mitt training and medicine ball workouts. The minimal pieces of equipment required are boxing gloves, a heavy bag and a jump rope.

Shadowboxing Warm-Up
(1 × 3-minute round)
Shadowboxing warms up your working muscles and prepares you mentally to work on the different bags and on target mitts. It also re-orientates you to the proper execution of the punches. Ensure there is adequate space to move around and throw your punches. If a mirror is available visually check to make sure your hands are held high, your body position is in the classic boxing stance, and your punches are crisp and clean. Always return the hands

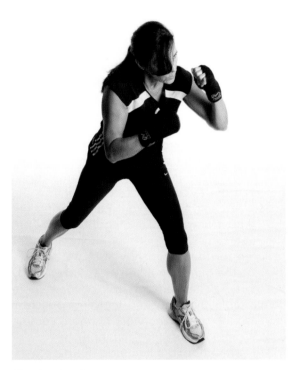

Shadowboxing.

Jump Rope
(3 × 3-minute rounds)

Start by jumping at a moderate pace keeping the footwork basic. As you become more experienced increase your jumping intensity. This can be accomplished by moving at a faster pace or by performing more intricate footwork, such as scissors, jumping jacks and even adding some sprints (see Chapter 5). The goal is to jump for 3 minutes straight, take a 1-minute break, and then repeat jumping two more times with a 1-minute break. This 1-minute break gives you time to stretch out tight calf muscles and reduce your breathing rate. Remember if you are having difficulty with continuous jumping or with executing the footwork, go back to the neutral move by placing both handles in one hand and rotate the rope at the side of your body. The goal of jumping rope is to condition your cardiovascular system, so you want to keep your heart rate elevated. Try to work at a perceived exertion of 7–9.

back to protect your chin. Add movement with your feet, head and body, keeping balanced and executing smoothly.

During the 1-minute rest, stretch out any muscles that feel tight (see Chapter 8 for specific exercises). Loosen up the shoulders, hip flexors and legs.

Shadowboxing
(1 × 3-minute round)

Throw your punches with a little more intensity. Move around and mix up the punches, moving forward and backward, and side-to-side. Develop smooth transitions both for your punches and your footwork. Balance is the key, and weight transfer should be effortless. After throwing a variety of straight punches, start to put together punch combinations. Focus on your punching technique until it becomes second nature. Get used to working for a full 3 minutes and pace yourself working at a perceived exertion of 5–6. (For more information on shadowboxing see Chapter 2.)

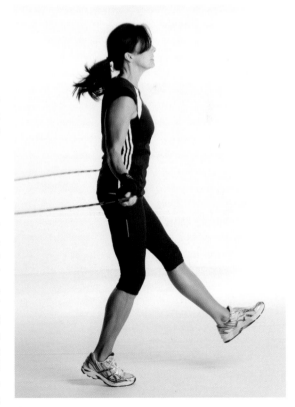

Jump rope.

Heavy Bag
(3 × 3-minute rounds)

Hit the bag for 3 minutes, and then take a 1-minute rest. Repeat this three times. Starting in the classic boxing stance with your hands up, throw left jabs as you move around the bag. Your left jab is your range finder, so start by throwing plenty of jabs to establish an effective distance from the bag and set a good punching pace. Keep busy, ensuring your movement and combinations flow easily and there are no long pauses between punches.

Start throwing one-twos (a left jab followed by a straight right). Visualize an opponent in front of you and keep moving. Simulate a body attack by bending the legs and lowering your body, hitting the mid-section of the bag. Find your rhythm and move naturally with the swinging motion of the bag. Find a consistent punching pace that you can continue with and persevere to the end of the round.

For the second and third rounds, work on 3- and 4-punch combinations (see Chapter 3). Keep moving during your 1-minute rest, walking around the bag reducing the heart rate slightly and planning your next round. Work at a perceived exertion of 7–9.

Focus Mitts
(2 × 3-minute rounds)

Partner Drill: When training on the focus mitts, concentrate on the proper execution of your punches and balanced footwork. Alternate the 3-minute rounds with your partner, taking turns punching and catching. You will also be getting a workout even when you catch the punches. Keep the combinations basic, starting with the straight punches. Establish a pattern of throwing many crisp jabs, continually moving in between the throws. The catcher controls the action and sets the workout pace, calling out the combinations and keeping the puncher in view at all times. The puncher must remember to listen for the commands from the catcher, execute the punch and then move away, ready for the next command. As you become more comfortable throwing and catching punches, increase the speed and work on more complicated combinations (see Chapter 4).

No-Partner Option: If you do not have partner, you can use the heavy bag as an alternate workout option.

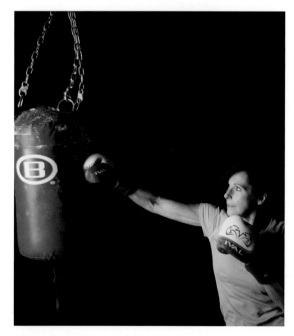

Heavy bag.

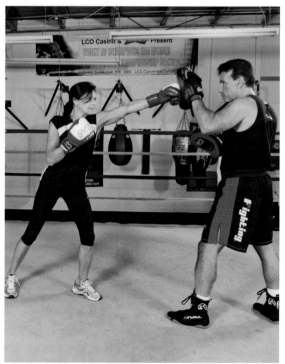

Focus mitts.

Heavy Bag Ladder Drill: This drill challenges your straight punching technique, foot movement, upper body conditioning and endurance. Try to complete this drill within 6 minutes.

Ladder 1: Throw 12 left jabs. Reduce the number of jabs you throw by 1 each time, continuing down the ladder until you throw just 1 jab. Take a 1-minute rest.

Ladder 2: Throw 12 one-two punch combinations (left jab–straight right). Reduce the number by 1 each time continuing down the ladder until you throw just 1 one-two punch combination (see Chapter 4).

Shadowboxing Cool-Down
(1 × 3-minute round)
Throw a variety of punches at 50–60 per cent effort. Even though you are not throwing as hard as you did during your workout it is still important to focus on the proper execution of the punches. Keep your feet moving side-to-side and front and back. Allow your heart rate to lower, catch your breath, and work at a perceived exertion of 3–4.

Core Strength Training
Select two to three medicine ball exercises to work your core muscles (see Chapter 7).

Sample sequence:

Medicine Ball Crunch: 10 to 20 repetitions with a 3–5kg (6–10lb) medicine ball. Perform 2 to 3 sets.

Overhead Pull-Up: 10 to 15 repetitions with a 3–5kg (6–10lb) medicine ball. Perform 2 to 3 sets.

Seated Bent Knee Tuck: 10 to 15 repetitions with a 3–5kg (6–10lb) medicine ball. Perform 2 to 3 sets.

Side Pullover Sit-Up: 10 to 15 repetitions with a 3–5kg (6–10lb) medicine ball. Perform 2 to 3 sets.

Shadowboxing cool-down.

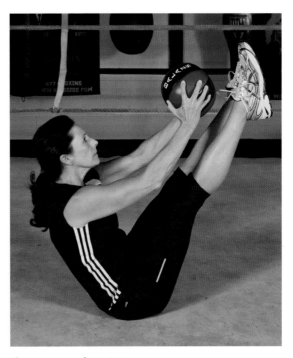
Core strength training.

Stretch

Select stretches for all the main muscle groups you have trained. Hold each stretch for 30–60 seconds (see Chapter 8).

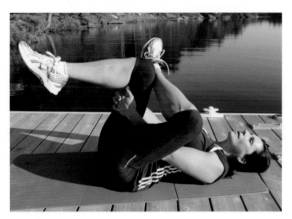

Stretch.

The Basic Workout Summary

(3-Day/Week Programme)

Shadowboxing Warm-Up

(1 × 3-minute round)
Shadowbox working on the basic punches. Focus on proper technique.

Shadowboxing

(1 × 3-minute round)
Add more movement while throwing more punches and combinations. Add more intent to the punches (see Chapter 2).

Jump Rope

(3 × 3-minute rounds)
Jump for 3 minutes straight, take a 1-minute break and repeat jumping for two more rounds with a 1-minute break in between (see Chapter 5).

Heavy Bag

(3 × 3-minute rounds)
Hit the bag for 3 minutes, and then take a 1-minute rest. Repeat this three times. Ensure your foot movement is balanced and your punch combinations flow (see Chapter 3).

Focus Mitts

(2 × 3-minute rounds)
Partner Drill: Alternate with your partner taking turns punching and catching (see Chapter 4).

No Partner Option: Heavy Bag Ladder Drill (6 minutes)

Ladder 1: Throw 12 left jabs, reducing down to 1 jab. Take a 1-minute rest.

Ladder 2: Throw 12 one-two punch combinations, reducing down to one-two punch combination (see Chapter 3).

Shadowboxing to Cool-Down

(1 × 3-minute round)
End with shadowboxing, punching with light intent. Reduce your heart rate.

Strength Training

Sample Sequence: Medicine Ball Crunch, Overhead Pull-Up, Seated Bent Knee Tuck, Side Pullover Sit-Up (see Chapter 7).

Final Stretch

Allow time to properly stretch out all the muscle groups and joint areas (see Chapter 8).

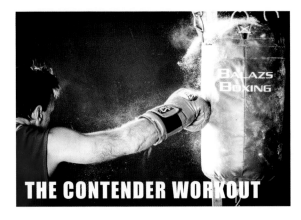

(5 Day/Week Programme)

The contender workout bumps up the intensity to a 5-day programme and requires a more serious commitment. The boxing training workout is performed 3 days a week and includes working on the heavy bag, jumping rope, shadow boxing, focus mitt training, double-end bag training and speed-bag work. In between your boxing training days are active rest days. On these days, roadwork and strength training with the medicine ball are performed. The roadwork and strength training will complement your boxing conditioning. Make a commitment to follow the contender workout for 12 weeks.

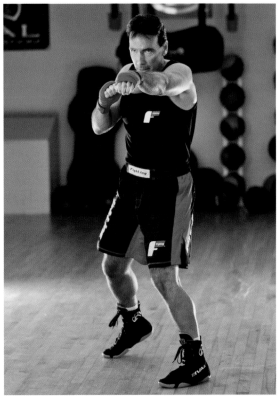

Shadowboxing.

BOXING WORKOUT...Day 1, 3, 5

(For example: Monday, Wednesday, and Friday)

Shadowboxing Warm-Up
(1 × 3 minute round)

Move around to warm up your muscles and throw easy punches to start. Focus on the execution of your punches, beginning with straight punches and then adding hooks and uppercuts. Continue moving for 3 minutes.

Rest for 1 minute, walking around and stretching out any muscles that feel tight. Loosen up the shoulders, hip flexors and legs (see Chapter 8).

Shadowboxing
(2 × 3 minute rounds)

Remember, shadowboxing is like being in the ring with an opponent. Visualize your opponent in front of you, move and punch, making use of the available floor space. Now that you have warmed up put more power behind your punches. Have a plan. Stay light on your feet and execute your punch combinations with balanced footwork. Practise mixing slips and ducks into your combinations, developing offensive and defensive moves. For the last round you may want to hold onto light hand weights (1–2kg, 0.5–1lb) punching at 60 per cent intensity (for more information on shadowboxing see Chapter 2). Work at a perceived exertion of 6–7.

Rest for 1 minute in between the shadowboxing rounds. Remember to allow your heart rate to come down slightly, keep moving around, and stretch out tight muscles.

Jump Rope
(9–12 minute continuous jumping)

Jump rope continuously for 9–12 minutes, mixing up the jumps and the intensity. For the first 2 minutes jump at a moderate pace, gradually increasing the speed and mixing up the footwork. Perform footwork patterns like the Ali shuffle, scissors and front crosses. Travel forward and backward and side-to-side, staying light on your feet (see Chapter 5). Work at a perceived exertion of 7–9.

Jump Rope Option: Another option is to perform the jump rope ladder drill in place of jumping continuously. Choose a number of jumps to start. For example, 400: count 400 jumps, and take a 30–60-second rest. Then reduce the number of jumps by 50 for each ladder: 350 jumps, rest; 300 jumps, rest; 250, rest and so forth (see Chapter 5).

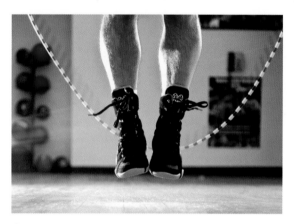

Jump rope.

Focus Mitts
(3 × 3-minute rounds)

If you are training with a partner alternate the 3 × 3-minute rounds with your partner, taking turns punching and catching. The puncher needs to focus on throwing fast accurate punches at the mitts, developing a smooth rhythm, and staying balanced. Catchers need to challenge their partner and set the pace. Remember working together as a team is the key when training on focus mitts. Incorporate a multitude of punch combinations that include slipping and ducking (see Chapter 4).

Ladder Punch Drill: Finish off your focus mitt training with the ladder punch drill by throwing the one-two punch combination at the focus mitts and then dropping and performing push-ups. Start with 8 one-twos and 8 push-ups for a total 36 punches/36 push-ups, working down to one of each (see Chapter 4).

If you do not have a partner to catch for you, go directly to the bag workouts.

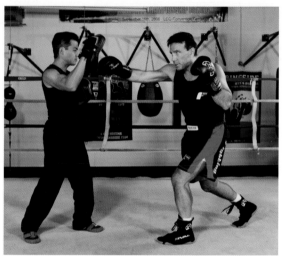

Focus mitts.

Heavy Bag
(4 × 3-minute rounds)

At the contender level you should be performing a greater variety of punches and punch combinations with fluid footwork and balanced body movement. Visualize an opponent in front of you as you punch. Add slips and feints staying light on your feet. Mix up your punches by throwing to the body area and head area of the bag. Always keep your hands up in the on-guard position as you move around the bag. Sustain a good punching pace for the entire 3 minutes of every round and use your 1-minute rest to recover between rounds. Keep moving during the 1-minute rest period and focus on the next round. Work at a perceived exertion of 7–9.

Complete three more heavy bag rounds, and finish off working on the bag by performing heavy bag sprints (see Chapter 3 if you want to substitute with a different drill).

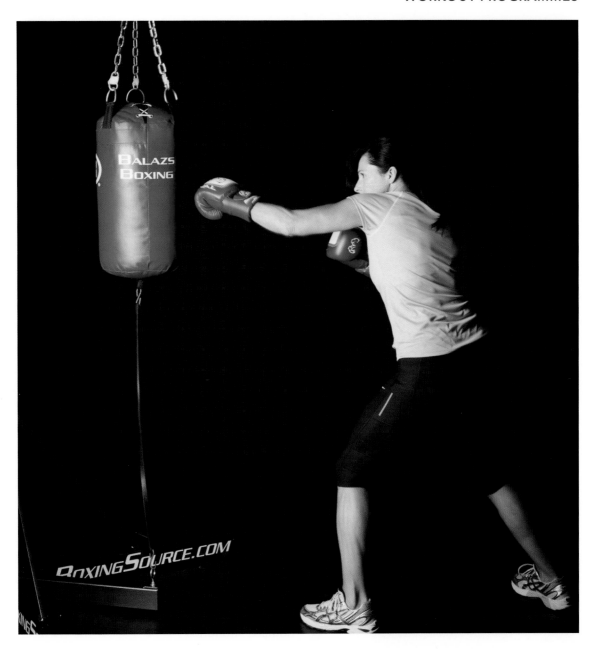

Heavy bag.

Heavy Bag Drill
Speed Sprints: Face the heavy bag straight on with both arms at an equal distance from the bag for the entire drill. Hit the bag continuously as fast as you can with a one-two, one-two rhythm. Keep your core held tight, weight centred through the balls of the feet, knees relaxed, and a steady breathing rate. Sprint for 25 seconds, rest for 25 seconds and repeat two more times. In the following weeks, increase your sprint time to 30 seconds, then 35 seconds, with the equivalent rest times. Always keep moving and walking around during the rest intervals. For your last sprint, work at a perceived exertion of 9–10. Take a 2-minute rest before working on the double-end bag.

Double-End Bag
(1 × 3 minute round)

If a double-end bag is available work on it for one round, perfecting the timing and speed of your punches, and the side-to-side movement of your head and body (see Chapter 3). Rest for 1 minute before hitting the speed bag.

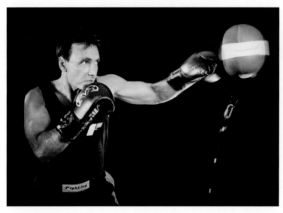

Double-end bag.

Speed Bag
(2 × 3 minute rounds)

Working out on the speed bag helps to develop hand-eye coordination and challenges your upper body endurance. Concentrate on striking the bag correctly to keep it moving smoothly (see Chapter 3). Rest for 1 minute between rounds.

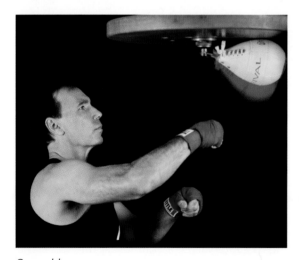

Speed bag.

Shadowboxing Cool-Down
(1 × 3 minute round)

Throw light punches working on technique and allow your heart rate to lower. Reduce your breathing rate and work at a perceived exertion of 3–4.

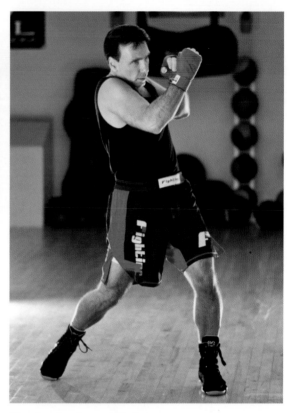

Shadowboxing cool-down.

Core Strength Training

Select two to three medicine ball exercises to work your core muscles (see Chapter 7). Sample Sequence:

Medicine Ball Crunch: 100 repetitions with a 3–5kg (6–10lb) medicine ball. If you prefer break up the repetitions into 2 sets of 50, with a 30-second break in between.

Medicine Ball Ab-Press: 15 repetitions with a medicine ball. Perform 2 to 3 sets.

V-Ups: 10 to 15 repetitions with a 3–4kg (6–8lb) medicine ball. Perform 2 to 3 sets.

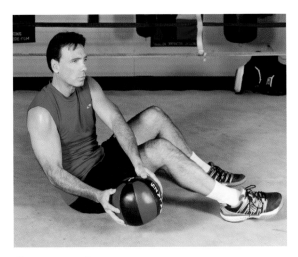

Core strength.

Stretch
Perform stretching exercises holding each stretch for 30–60 seconds (see Chapter 8).

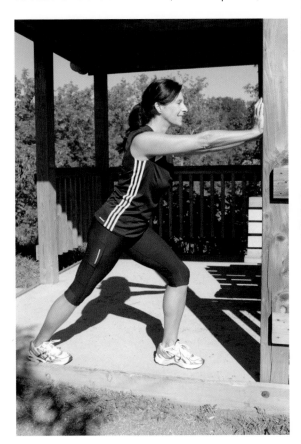

Stretch.

ROADWORK AND STRENGTH TRAINING... Days 2, 4
(for example Tuesday and Thursday)

Roadwork
Depending on your fitness level and running ability, run continuously for 30–45 minutes. Start with a warm-up by jogging or running slowly for 1km (0.6 mile). Run at a moderate pace and at a perceived exertion rate of 6–7. If you are an experienced runner vary the tempo of your running pace from time to time. Work at a higher intensity for a specified distance or time and then return to the moderate pace (see Chapter 6).

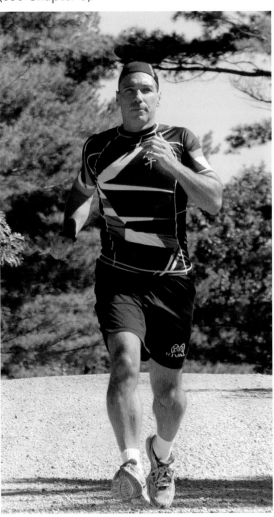

Roadwork.

Strength Training

Select 6 to 9 medicine ball exercises to work your full body, upper body, core and lower body (see Chapter 7). Sample sequence:

Full Body

Woodchopper: 10 to 12 repetitions, holding a 3–4kg (6–8lb) medicine ball. Perform two to 3 sets.

Medicine Ball Burpees: 12 to 15 repetitions. Select a medicine ball that is larger in size to give you a more stable base. Perform 2 to 3 sets.

Upper Body:

Staggered Push-Ups: 10 to 12 repetitions. Select a medicine ball that is larger in size to give you a more stable base. Perform 2 sets.

Core

Side Pullover Sit-Up: 10 to 15 repetitions with a 3–5kg (6–10lb) medicine ball. Perform 1 to 2 sets.

V-Ups: 10 to 15 repetitions with a 3–4kg (6–8lb) medicine ball. Perform 2 to 3 sets.

Medicine Ball Ab-Press: 15 repetitions, holding a 3–5kg (6–10lb) medicine ball. Perform 3 sets.

Medicine Ball Plank: Hold for 30 seconds, increasing to 60 seconds. Perform 2 to 3 sets.

Lower Body

Power Squats: 10 to 15 repetitions holding a 3–5kg (6–10lb) medicine ball. Perform 1 to 2 sets.

Forward Lunges: 10 to 20 repetitions for each leg holding a 4–7kg (8–15lb) medicine ball. Perform 2 to 3 sets.

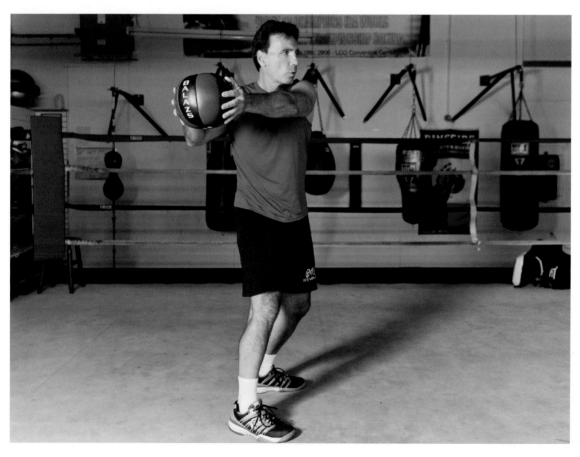

Strength training.

Stretch

Select stretches for all the main muscle groups you have trained. Hold each stretch for 30–60 seconds (see Chapter 8).

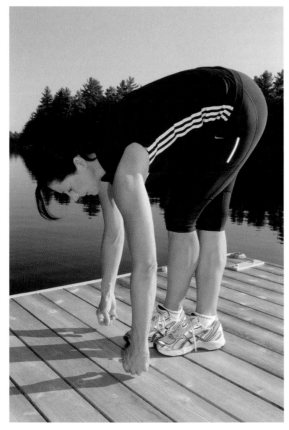

Stretch.

The Contender Workout Summary

(5-Day/Week Programme – for 12 Weeks)

Shadowboxing Warm-Up

(1 × 3 minute round)

Warm up your muscles and throw easy punches to start.

Shadowboxing

(2 × 3 minute rounds)

Increase the intensity of your punches (see Chapter 2).

Jump Rope

(9–12 minutes)

Jump rope continuously for 9–12 minutes, mixing up your footwork (see Chapter 5).

Focus Mitts

(3 × 3-minute rounds)

Alternate catching and punching rounds with your partner. Include a multitude of punch combinations that include slipping and ducking (see Chapter 4).

Focus Mitt Drill

Ladder Punch Drill: Perform 8 one-twos and 8 push-ups for a total 36 punches/36 push-ups, working down to 1 of each (see Chapter 4).

If you do not have a partner go directly to the bag workouts.

Heavy Bag

(4 × 3-minute rounds)

Challenge yourself by throwing a wide variety of punch combinations. Sustain a good punching pace for the entire 3 minutes of every round (see Chapter 3).

Heavy Bag Drill

Speed Sprints: Sprint for 25 seconds, rest for 25 seconds and repeat two more times. Increase your sprint time to 30 seconds, then 35 seconds, with the equivalent rest time.

Sprint 1	25 seconds (rest 25 seconds)
Sprint 2	25 seconds (rest 25 seconds)
Sprint 3	25 seconds (rest 25 seconds)

Double-End Bag

(1 × 3 minute round)

Work one round on the double-end bag, perfecting the timing and speed of your punches and the side-to-side movement of your head and body (see Chapter 3).

Speed Bag

(2 × 3 minute rounds)

Work out on the speed bag maintaining a smooth rhythm and fast pace (see Chapter 3).

Shadowboxing Cool-Down
(1 × 3 minute round)
Throw light punches working on technique. Allow your heart rate to lower.

Strength Training
(4–6 minutes)
Medicine Ball Crunch, Medicine Ball Ab Press, V-Ups (see Chapter 7).

Stretch
Allow time to properly stretch out all the muscle groups and joint areas (see Chapter 8).

Roadwork
(30–45 minutes)
Start by jogging at an easy pace for 1km. Run at a moderate pace for 30 to 45 minutes. Include interval training (see Chapter 6).

Strength Training
Perform 6–9 exercises.
Woodchopper, Medicine Ball Burpee, Staggered Push-up, Side Pullover Sit-up, V-Ups, Medicine Ball Ab Press, Medicine Ball Plank, Power Squats, Forward Lunges (see Chapter 7).

Final Stretch
Allow time to properly stretch out all the muscle groups and joint areas (see Chapter 8).

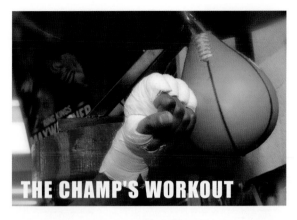

THE CHAMP'S WORKOUT

(6 Days/Week Programme)

For the champ's workout, an extra day of training is added for a total of 6 days per week over a 12-week period. The intensity level is increased and a focused commitment is required. Perform the boxing workout 3 times per week, and on the alternate active rest days perform roadwork and strength training with the medicine ball. Take advantage of the one day off to recover from the six days of training.

The boxing workout includes the heavy bag, jump rope, shadow boxing, focus mitts, double-end bag, speed bag and strength training with the medicine ball. The active rest days include roadwork, sprints and strength training with the medicine ball.

BOXING WORKOUT

(Perform on alternate days. For example: Monday, Wednesday, and Friday.)

Shadowboxing Warm-Up
(1 × 3-minute round)
Throw light punches to start, focusing on proper execution. Begin with straight punches and then add hooks and uppercuts. Continue moving for 3 minutes.

Shadowboxing
(2 × 3-minute rounds)
Now that you have warmed up, put more power and intensity behind your punches.

Move and throw punches at your virtual opponent. Practise offensive and defensive moves (see Chapter 2).

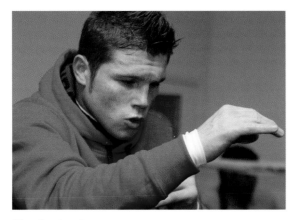

Shadowboxing.

Jump Rope
(Continuous for 15-20 minutes)

For your jump rope training session, start by jumping at a moderate pace for the first few minutes to warm up your joints and muscles and to set your jumping rhythm. Challenge yourself by adding a variety of footwork and rope moves. Perform double unders, crossovers, and speed sprints within your training. Finish off with a 2–3 minute cool-down, reducing the pace of your jumps (see Chapter 5).

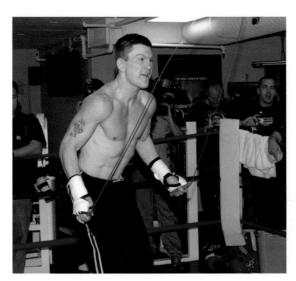

Jump rope.

Focus Mitt Drill
(4 × 3-minute rounds)

Focus mitt training allows you to bring all of your fitness boxing skills into play. This dynamic training sharpens your punching skills, defensive moves, reflexes and balance, and develops upper body strength and endurance. At the champ's level you want to throw a wide a variety of punch combinations and at a higher level of intensity. If you are proficient at executing the advanced combinations described in Chapter 4, you may want to develop your own punch combinations. When creating your own combinations ensure a logical sequence is followed and that each punch smoothly sets up the next punch or movement.

Focus Mitt Sprints: This rapid-fire series of straight punches, hooks, uppercuts, slipping, and ducking challenges and develops your cardio endurance. Maintain a quick pace and execute the punches with proper technique. Begin with 20-second sprints and increase the time increment to 30–40 second sprints. Repeat the sprint sequence twice and then switch roles with your training partner (see Chapter 4).

Sprint 1

Straight lefts and rights	20 seconds
Left and right hooks	20 seconds
Left and right uppercuts	20 seconds
Slipping side-to-side	20 seconds

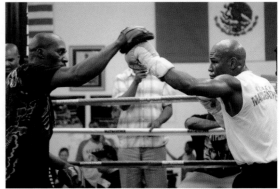

Focus mitts.

Sprint 2

Straight lefts and rights	20 seconds
Left and right hooks	20 seconds
Left and right uppercuts	20 seconds
Ducking under	20 seconds

It is important to modify focus mitt workouts to each individual's ability and skill level. This is accomplished by adapting the intensity level and the punch sequencing of the drill.

Heavy Bag
(5 × 3-minute rounds)

Train on the heavy bag as though you are facing an actual opponent in the ring, constantly moving while throwing punch combinations. Include feints, slips, and ducks into the mix and visualize deceiving your opponent in order to set up a punch opportunity (see Chapter 2). Adding these subtle movements adds another element to your heavy bag training. Coordinate your footwork and punches with the swinging motion of the bag. Remember real boxing matches do not have long periods of inactivity. Throw plenty of punches and keep moving to emulate real fight situations. Move around during the 1-minute rest period and plan your next round. Work at a perceived exertion of 7-9.

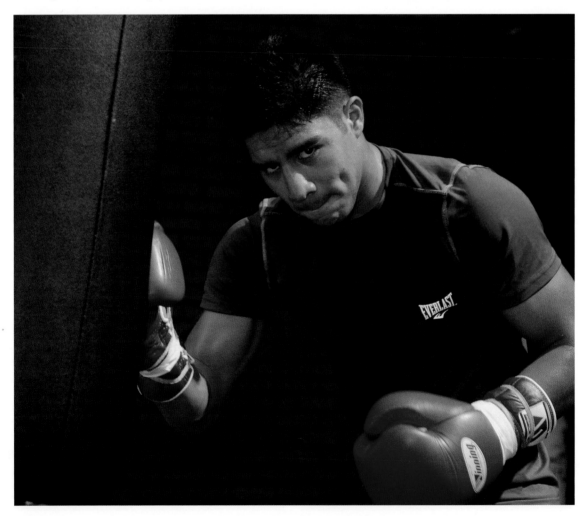

Heavy bag.

Theme Your Rounds

When hitting the heavy bag, theme your rounds by emulating different boxing styles. For example for one round simulate the style of boxers who have incredible footwork and hand speed, such as Muhammad Ali and Sugar Ray Leonard. The challenge is to constantly move and change direction while firing off long-range punches. In your next round emulate the style of a close-range, inside fighter. Champion Gennady Golovkin continually moves forward to land powerful hooks and uppercuts. Working on different fighting styles allows you to get the maximum out of your fitness boxing workout.

Heavy Bag Drill
(1 × 3-minute round)

Dirty 30s: Move around the bag and execute a series of fast punches for 30 seconds. Now face the bag straight on, punching and running on the spot lifting your knees high. For the last 30 seconds return to the boxing stance, and go all-out like you are trying to knock out your opponent. Complete the sequence twice without stopping to complete the 3-minute round (see Chapter 3). Working at a perceived exertion of 8-9. Take a 1–2 minute rest before hitting the double-end bag.

Double-End Bag
(2 × 3-minute rounds)

Throw punch combinations and slips ensuring you are in a balanced position reacting to the quick movement and the rebound action of the double-end bag. Develop your timing and rhythm, constantly moving and firing rapid-fire punches (see Chapter 3). Rest for 1 minute in between rounds and before hitting the speed bag.

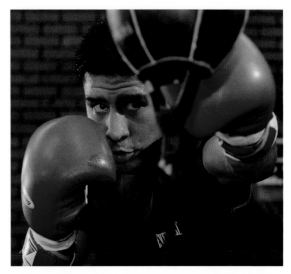

Double-end bag.

Speed Bag
(6–8 minutes)

Challenge your upper body endurance by hitting the speed bag at a fast pace for 6-8 minutes. Rest for 1 minute before moving onto the shadowboxing.

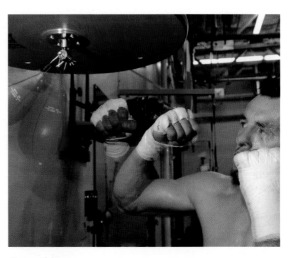

Speed bag.

Shadowboxing Cool-Down
(1 × 3-minute round)

Slow down your movements and reduce your breathing rate. By the end of the cool-down round you should be at a perceived exertion of 3-4.

Core Strength – Medicine Ball

Select two medicine ball strength exercises to train your core region (see Chapter 7). Sample sequence:

Medicine Ball Cycle: 30 to 40 repetitions, holding a 3–5kg (6–10lb) medicine ball. Perform 2 sets.

Roll-Up and Knee Tuck: 10 to 15 repetitions with a 3–4kg (6–8lb) medicine ball. Perform 2 to 3 sets.

Core Strength – Focus Mitts
(2 minutes)

Focus Mitt Abdominal Punch-Up Drill: complete 2 sets of 30-second straight punches, hooks and uppercuts (see Chapter 4).

If you have a partner perform focus mitts abs. If not select another core exercise from Chapter 7.

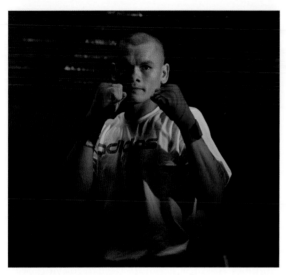

Shadowboxing cool-down.

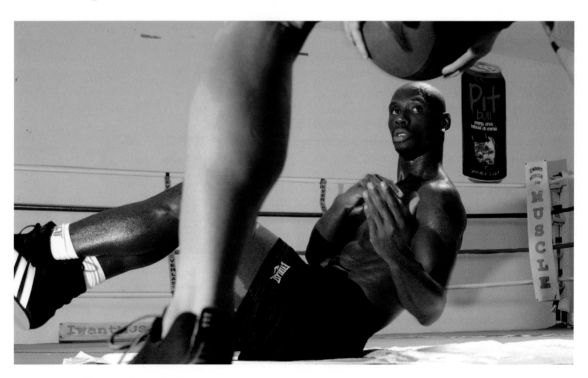

Core strength – medicine ball.

Stretch

Perform stretching exercises holding each stretch for 30-60 seconds (see Chapter 8).

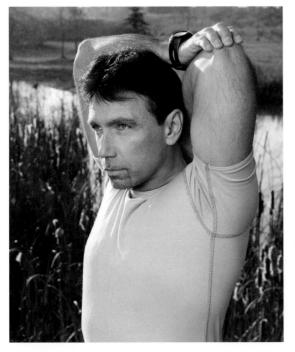

Stretches.

ROADWORK AND STRENGTH TRAINING

(Perform on alternate days. For example: Tuesday, Thursday, and Saturday.)

Roadwork

Perform your roadwork training first. Include intervals, sprints and an occasional aerobic longer run (see Chapter 6).

Intervals: Jog for 1km at a moderate pace to warm up. Pick up the pace and run for 200m or 400m (or 1-2 minutes) at a perceived exertion of 6-7. Now bump up the intensity for the next interval and run a distance of 200m or 400m (or 1-2 minutes) at a perceived exertion to 8-9. Repeat the intervals six times. Finish off with an easy 1-2km jog.

Distance Sprints: One day a week, include sprint work during the interval sessions.

Sample Routine: Warm up by jogging for 400m. Sprint for 200m, at a perceived exertion level of 9-10. Keep up this running intensity for the entire distance and then jog or walk back (200 metres) to your starting point. Repeat the sprint six times. Jog for 800m to cool down after your last interval.

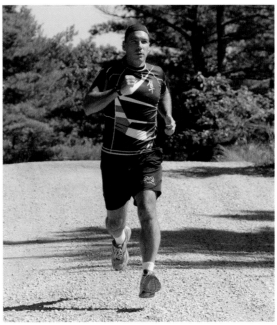

Roadwork.

Strength Training

Select 8 to 12 medicine ball exercises to work your full body, upper body, core and lower body (see Chapter 7). Sample sequence:

Full Body

Rock 'n Roll: 10 to 12 repetitions, holding a 3-4kg (6-8lb) medicine ball. Perform 2 to 3 sets.

Mountain Climber: 12 to15 repetitions or for 20-40 seconds using a larger sized medicine ball. Perform 2 to 3 sets.

Upper Body

The Boxer's Push-Up: 8 to 12 repetitions using a larger sized medicine ball. Perform 2 to 3 sets.

Standing Medicine Ball Twist: 8 to 12 repetitions with a 3-5kg (6-10lb) medicine ball. Perform 1 to 3 sets.

Core

Overhead Pull-Ups: 10 to 15 repetitions with a 3-5kg (6-10lb) medicine ball. Perform 2 to 3 sets.

Medicine Ball Ab-Press: 15 repetitions, holding a 3-5kg (6-10lb) medicine ball. Perform 2 to 3 sets.

Side Pullover Sit-Up: 10 to 15 repetitions with a 3-5kg (6-10lb) medicine ball. Perform 2 sets.

Roll-Up and Knee Tuck: 10 to 15 repetitions with a 3-4kg (6-8lb) medicine ball. Perform 2 to 3 sets.

Seated Bent Knee Tuck: 10 to 15 repetitions with a 3-5kg (6-10lb) medicine ball. Perform 1 to 3 sets.

Lower Body

180s: 12 to 15 repetitions or for 20–40 seconds, using a 3-4kg (6-8lb) medicine ball. Perform 1 to 2 sets.

Forward Lunges: 10 to 20 repetitions for each leg holding a 4-7kg (8-15lb) medicine ball. Perform 2 to 3 sets.

Power Squats: 10 to 15 repetitions holding a 3-5kg (6-12lb) medicine ball. Perform 1 to 2 sets.

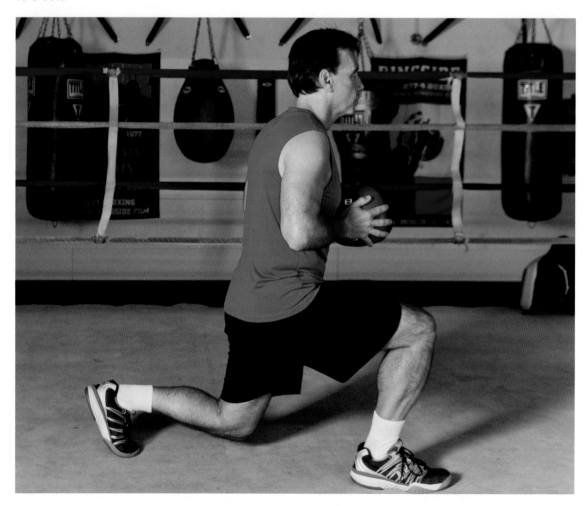

Strength training.

Stretch

Select stretches for all the main muscle groups you have trained. Hold each stretch for 30–60 seconds (see Chapter 8).

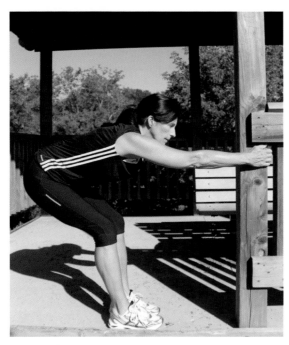

Stretch.

The Champ's Workout Summary

(6 Days/Week Programme – for 12 Weeks)

Shadowboxing Warm-Up

(1 × 3-minute round)
Gradually warm up and prepare for your workout.

Shadowboxing

(2 × 3-minute rounds)
Pick up the pace. Move and throw punches at your virtual opponent (see Chapter 2).

Jump Rope

(Continuous for 15–20 minutes)
Challenge yourself by adding a variety of footwork and rope moves. Finish off with a 2–3 minute cool-down (see Chapter 5).

Focus Mitts

(4 × 3-minute rounds)
Throw a wide a variety of punch combinations, at a high level of intensity (see Chapter 4).

Sprint 1

Straight lefts and rights	30 seconds
Left and right hooks	30 seconds
Left and right uppercuts	30 seconds
Slipping side-to-side	30 seconds

Sprint 2

Straight lefts and rights	30 seconds
Left and right hooks	30 seconds
Left and right uppercuts	30 seconds
Ducking under	30 seconds

Heavy Bag

(5 × 3-minutes rounds)
Constantly move while throwing punch combinations including feints, slips and ducks into the mix (see Chapter 2).

Heavy Bag Drill

(1 × 3-minute round)
Dirty 30s: Box for 30 seconds, high knees and punch for 30 seconds and power punch for 30 seconds. Repeat the sequence to complete the 3-minute round (see Chapter 3).

Double-End Bag

(2 × 3 minute rounds)
Throw punch combination and slips (see Chapter 3).

Speed Bag

(6–8 minutes)
Strike the speed bag at a fast pace for 6–8 minutes.

Shadowboxing Cool-Down

(1 × 3-minute round)
Throw your punches lightly to cool down.

Core Strength: Medicine Ball

Medicine Ball Cycle and Roll-Up and Knee Tuck.

Core Strength: Focus Mitts

Focus Mitt Abdominal Punch-Up Drill (see Chapter 4).

If you have a partner perform focus mitts abs. If not select another core exercise from Chapter 7.

Stretch

Allow time to properly stretch out all the muscle groups and joint areas (see Chapter 8).

Roadwork

Jog at an easy pace for 1km to warm-up. Perform interval work (distance 200–400m or timed at 1–2 minutes) Include timed sprints, distance sprints or hill sprints. Finish with an easy run (see Chapter 6).

Strength Training

Perform 10 to 12 exercises (Chapter 7).
Rock 'n Roll, Mountain Climber, Upper Body, The Boxer's Push-Up, Standing Medicine Ball Twist, Overhead Pull-Ups, Medicine Ball Ab-Press, Side Pullover Sit-Up, Roll-Up and Knee Tuck, Seated Bent Knee Tuck, 180s, Forward Lunges, Power Squats.

Final Stretch

Allow time to properly stretch out all the muscle groups and joint areas (see Chapter 8).

Fitness Boxing at a Private Club

More and more gyms are offering fitness boxing classes for small groups, as well as private instruction with a certified trainer. If you are searching for a fitness boxing class look for a facility that has the basic boxing equipment, such as heavy bags, double-end bags and speed bags. Ensure there is sufficient space to jump rope, work on focus mitts with a partner, and mirrors to check your punch execution and movement.

Work with trainers who are certified with a recognized boxing/fitness association. Take time to watch a training session before you make your decision to participate. A trainer should be knowledgeable and approachable, and give clear, positive and direct instruction and feedback. A good trainer will bring out the best in you and provide a fun, safe, and effective workout that meets all of your fitness goals.

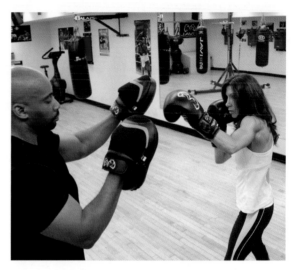

Working with a partner – focus mitts.

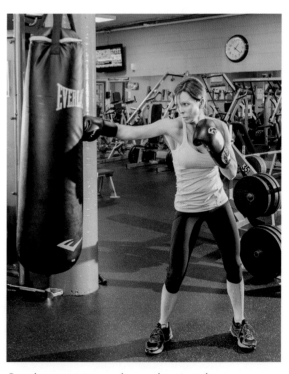

Southpaw stance – heavy bag workout.

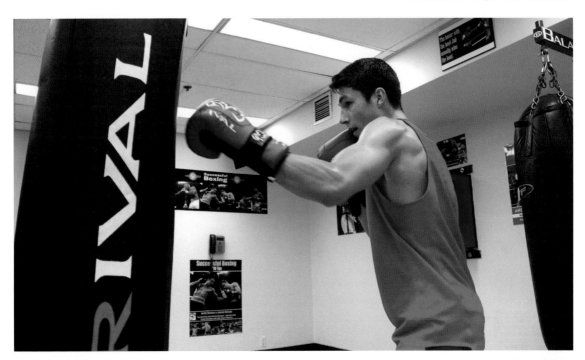

Put passion into your workouts.

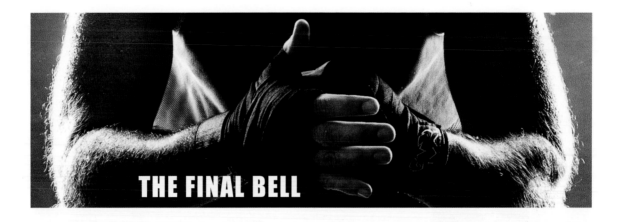

THE FINAL BELL

The development of this book was inspired by the great boxing champions and trainers, past and present. Great boxers show a passion and a dedication to perfecting their craft and to achieving superb physical conditioning. They know that everything meaningful in life results from hard work and putting in an honest effort.

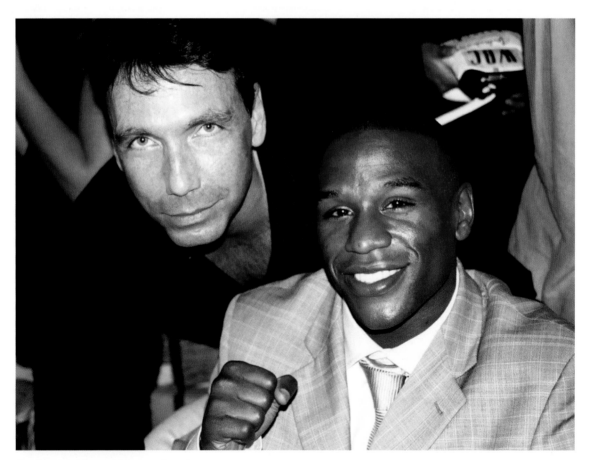

Andy with Floyd Mayweather Jr.

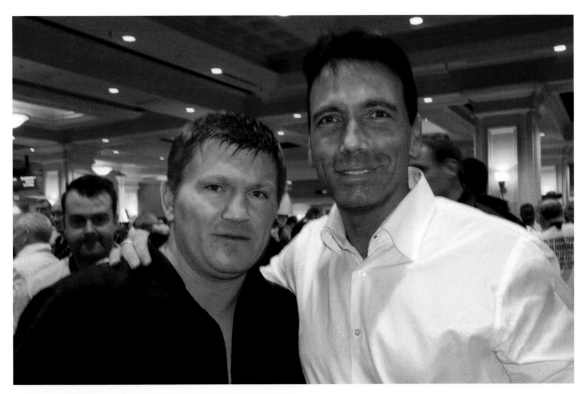

Andy with Ricky Hatton.

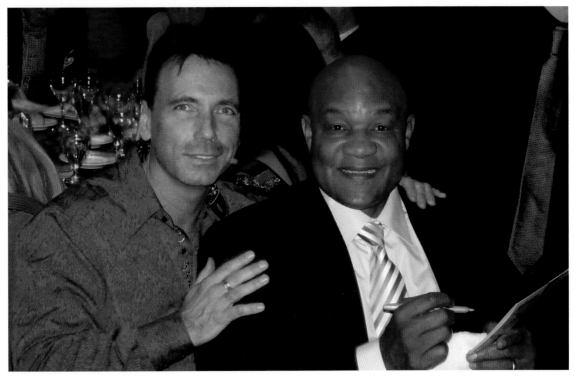

Andy with George Foreman.

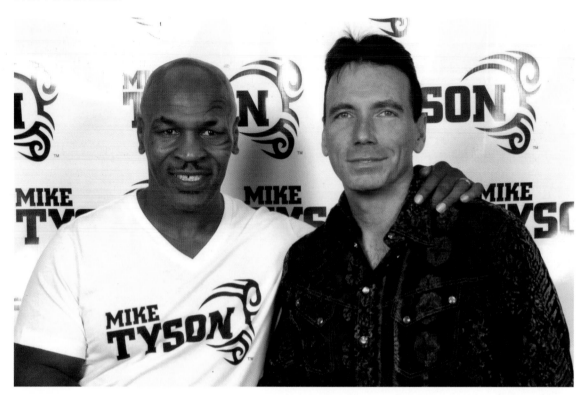

Andy with Mike Tyson.

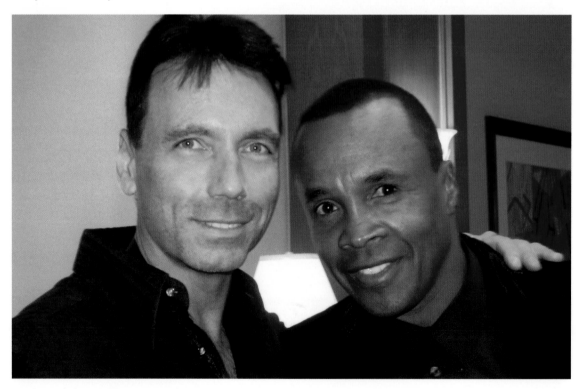

Andy with Sugar Ray Leonard.

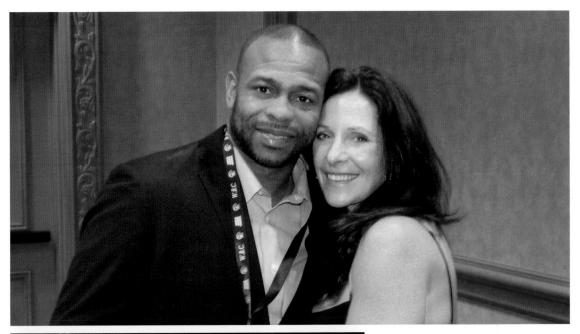

Jamie with Roy Jones Jr.

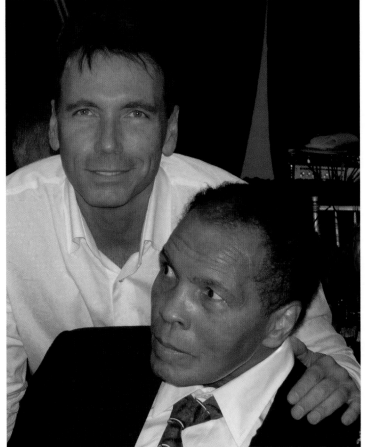

Success comes from doing little things correctly, day in and day out. Our advice is to continue to practise and improve, working the fundamentals, and strive to get better each and every day. We hope the information provided in the book will provide you with years of enjoyable, challenging and effective workouts.

Andy with Muhammad Ali.

INDEX